Evidence-Based Tai Chi for Rehabilitation and Wellness: A System of Balance for Clinical Practice

Mirella Veras, PhD

DEDICATION

This book is dedicated to my family for their constant encouragement, love, inspiration and support. A special dedication to my daughter, Rayne Maria Bastien. She has been my inspiration and motivation for continuing to improve my knowledge and move forward to new discoveries in life. She has made me stronger, better and more fulfilled than I could have ever imagined. I love you to Pluto and back

Table of Contents

ABOUT THE AUTHOR

Dr. Mirella Veras, PT, PhD, M.Sc. Registered physiotherapist with a PhD in Population Health (University of Ottawa, Canada), Master degree in Public Health/Epidemiology (Universidade Federal do Ceara, Brazil) and a postdoctoral in Rehabilitation Sciences from the University of Montreal, Canada. She has many years of experience as a physiotherapist, including as a clinician, consultant, professor and coordinator of health services. She works as a physiotherapist with people who have physical, mental health and/or behavioural challenges. She has a special interest in neuromusculoskeletal and women's health. She is a certified instructor for Tai Chi for Arthritis, Diabetes and Fall Prevention.

ACKNOWLEDGMENTS

I thank God for all the blessings He bestowed upon my life.
I have great pleasure in acknowledging my gratitude to Shane, for all of his love and support and for standing beside me throughout my career and writing this book. I am grateful to all my Tai Chi teachers and mentors for their wisdom and experience.
I would like to express my gratitude to Maureen Eagle Aalders, physiotherapist with many years of experience as a clinician and educator, for editing and providing many valuable comments that improved the presentation and contents of this book. She has sparked many interesting and good-spirited discussions relating to the System of Balance concepts and ideas. We worked together to develop the definition of the System of Balance presented in this book.
I would like to express my special appreciation and thanks to Angela Morrison for her brilliant comments and suggestions for our Tai Chi groups and photography of the exercises. I thank her for all the assistance she has provided me with practical suggestions and helpful advice for adapting Tai Chi to people with mental health and behavioural challenges.
I would like to thank Tracie Sarsfield-Turner, Director of Clinical Services of the Kings Regional Rehabilitation Centre, who has provided me support and encouragement in pursuing Tai Chi education and work at the Kings Regional Rehabilitation Centre in Waterville, NS, Canada.
I would like to thank Bruno Wendel Costa dos Santos for the graphic design for the pictures and Tai Chi Logomak design.
Words cannot express how grateful I am to my clients and patients for their support and for the confidence that they have placed in me. I would like to assure them that I do not take this confidence for granted.

"Mastering others is strength. Mastering yourself is true power."
— Lao Tzu

FOREWORD

Dr. Mirella Veras and I have an emergent relationship through which we share a common interest in exploring the enhancement of well-being to reach one's full potential – all people, all potential! The shared experience has been Tai Chi and our working relationships with people who have varying abilities. While some folks are capable of self-direction, others require gentle nudging or perhaps even direct guidance.

"Every human has four endowments –
self awareness, conscience, independent will and creative imagination.
These give us the ultimate human freedom…
The power to choose, to respond, to change."

(Stephen Covey)

Dr. Veras is a passionate believer in the power of improving all aspects of "self" employing the principles of Tai Chi – whether it be through the traditional sequences of movement in its various styles or through her distinctive "postures" presented in this manual. She brings a pioneering spirit to this book and is sure to capture your attention. As a newcomer, it may just spark your fascination for Tai Chi. As a veteran, it may bolster your regard for Tai Chi and its role in "wholeness".
The favourable health and wellness benefits of Tai Chi have been researched and are well-documented. There is a wide variety of printed material outlining the history of Tai Chi, exploring its essence, and providing instruction in Tai Chi forms and sequences. This book, however, is a unique and alluring educational gem! Dr. Veras does indeed provide an overview of the origins of Tai Chi as well as commentary on some of its nuances, but she has cleverly created postures incorporating principles of Tai Chi. Dr. Veras utilized her knowledge of physiotherapy as well as her rekindled love of Tai Chi to give birth to these specific movements designed to enhance one's overall well-being. These "one of a kind" postures can be considered as direct intervention for "imbalances" or simply movement for wellness.

The postures can be separated into their components dependent upon the participant's skill level.

Dr. Veras has devised these postures – each having their own title, as a means of integrating principles of Tai Chi into human movement. Trying to assimilate the many facets of Tai Chi may seem daunting. This book can help you get started on your journey. Even those who are well-seasoned, may find a hidden treasure and will say that our journey "evolves" and there is always potential for new growth.

This book is certain to delight. Move through it slowly, enjoy the heightened physical ability, the enlightenment that is sure to blossom and getting to know yourself better ….. Repeat!

Whether you are a novice or a master in Tai Chi….

" Start where you are.
Use what YOU have.
Do what you can."

(Arthur Ashe)

Maureen Eagle Aalders, Physiotherapist
Cambridge Station, NS (Summer 2018)

Maureen Eagle Aalders is a physiotherapist who has 35 years of experience – most of which she has had the distinct pleasure of working with and learning from those who present with "life challenges" in areas of cognitive, physical and/or behavioural realms. She has also been an educator of select health care groups on the topic of safe and healthy body movement. Ms. Eagle Aalders has received certification through the Tai Chi for Health Institute in the Tai Chi for Arthritis and Fall Prevention program created by Dr. Paul Lam.

DISCLAIMER

No part of this book may be reproduced or transmitted in any form or by any means, electronic or mechanical, including photocopying, recording or by any information storage and retrieval system, without written permission from the author.

The information provided within this book is for general informational purposes only. This book is not intended to be a substitute for the medical or health professional advice of a licensed health professional. The reader should consult with their health professional in any matters relating to personal health. Before beginning any new exercise program, it is recommended that you seek medical advice from your personal physician, physiotherapist or health professional.

1 CHAPTER
HISTORY OF TAI CHI

"In all changes exists Tai Chi, which causes the two opposites in everything."

(The Book of Changes)

The term "Tai Chi" was first mentioned during the Zhou Dynasty (11th century-221 BC), in the Book of Changes, as described below (Koo, 2017):

"In all changes exists Tai Chi, which causes the two opposites in all things. The two opposites cause the four seasons, and the four seasons cause the eight natural phenomena." (Mena Koo-The Dance of the Tai Chi.p.39-40)

Tai chi (taiji), short for T'ai chi ch'üan, or Taijiquan (pinyin: tàijíquán; 太极拳) is an ancient Chinese form of exercise originally created as an internal Chinese martial art practiced for both self-defence and health benefits (Man-ch'ing, 1993). The term "internal" martial arts refers to martial arts with a focus on the spiritual, mental or qi-related aspects, as opposed to an "external" method that emphasises the physical application of the force. While the internal martial arts focuses on the training of chi through exercises like QiGong (philosophy of the forces yin and yang), the external martial arts emphasises the training of physical and muscular strength. However, many experts in the field believe that there is no such thing as an "internal art" or an "external art". There are individuals that practice an art "internally" and others practice the art "externally" (Beta, May 2018).The history of Tai Chi is mixed with legendary and historical descriptions of Tai Chi family practitioners. The legendary history begins from Buddha in India, also known as Siddhārtha Gautama, the old ancient time (500 or 600 BC). Some believe that Buddha lifted a lotus flower and smiled to everyone in a meeting on the Mount Lengjia. At this time, no one knew the meaning except for one person, JiaYe, disciple of Buddha, who also smiled to Buddha. Then, the Buddha announced to everybody: "I have a treasure, like a secret mountain, which is real but without any appearance, now I give it to JiaYe the Great." He said that "the treasure is passed from heart to heart directly, and this is also the case in the following generation when they pass the treasure of Zen. " (The history of Tai Chi, 2018). The treasure was passed from Zen to DaMo who left India and went to China (Liang Dynasty, before Tang Dynasty in China). DaMo met the Emperor and settled down in Shao-Lin Temple. He initiated the Chinese Zen and contributed to the Shao-Lin

Kongfu, although it is a method of fighting, it also helps individuals to improve their mind/spirit (The history of Tai Chi, 2018).

There is also another legendary history that Tai Chi was developed by a Taoist Priest named Zhang San Feng (1279-1368), a great master of Shao-Lin Chuan from a temple in China's Wu Dong Mountains. It says that he had a dream where God taught him how to fight. The priest observed a white crane preying on a snake, and imitated their movements to create the Tai Chi martial art style (Stanford University, 2018) (Galante, 1981). He was inspired by that scene where he noticed the softness, yielding and pliability of the animal's movements. Then, he created the Wu Tang School of meditation and martial arts (Galante, 1981).

Other references about Tai Chi indicate that the Li Family Manual is a valuable resource about the Tai Chi classics. The Li Family Manual has thirteen movements which are very similar to Tajiquan or Tai Chi. Li Chunmao learned the art of Tai Chi with thirteen movements and he seems to be the first person who practiced Tai Chi (Christensen, 2016).

The earliest version and pre-cursor of Tai Chi is credited to a physician, Hua-tu'o (the period of the Three Kingdoms: 220 to 265 AD) who taught a system he called Wu-chi chih his (the 'movements of the five creatures': tiger, deer, bear, ape and birds). He believed in a system of imitating the movements of these animals to exercise each joint in the body and help digestion and circulation for a long and healthy life (The History of Tai Chi, 2018).

The history after Chang San-Feng is not clear with many contradictory versions and dates. There are other martial arts similar to Tai Chi such as sanshiqi (三世七), xiantianquan (先天拳), and Xiaojiutian (小九天), and houtianfa (後天法). The martial art Houtianfa (後天法) was created by Hujingzi during the Liang Dynasty and includes the "eight directions" methods that are the core elements of Tai Chi Chuan. There is also another version that Chen Wangting (1600-1680 C.E.), a retired military officer created at the end of the Ming Dynasty - Tai Chi Chuan, and passed it on to descendants (Taichicentral.com, 2018).

2 CHAPTER

THE PHILOSOPHY AND PRINCIPLES OF TAI CHI

"It does not matter how slow you go as long as you do not stop"
Confucius

The philosophy of Tai Chi is based on the Taoist philosophy where the principles of softness, centeredness, yielding, balance, suppleness, slowness and rootedness are all elements present in Taoism. The term Tai Chi is an abbreviation for Tai Chi Chuan where Tai Chi in Mandarin means "The Supreme Ultimate Boxing System" and "Chuan" means "fist" and "fighting system". It also means "control" or "self-control". The name Tai Chi Chuan derives from Taoism (Galante, 1981). The martial art of Tai Chi is based on thirteen principles, where five of them refer to the footwork methodology responsible for moving the feet and body smoothly and with stability (step forward, step backward, gaze (that is, focus your intention toward and move) to the left, gaze to the right, and central equilibrium) (Frantzis, 2018).

The Tai Chi classics refer to circles (Yin and Yang) and the thirteen basic movements which relate to the Five phases and the Eight trigrams (Christensen, 2016). The "Five Phases" are Wood (木 mù), Fire (火 huǒ), Earth (土 tǔ), Metal (金 jīn), and Water (水 shuǐ). They are also known as Wu Xing, Five Elements, the Five Agents, the Five Movements, Five Processes, the Five Steps/Stages and the Five Planets of important gravity: Jupiter-木, Saturn-土, Mercury-水, Venus-金, Mars-火 (Dr Zai, 2015).

The Five-element theory (475-221 BC) is one of the most important representations of this unique philosophical system. Chinese ancients recognized that wood, fire, earth, metal, and water are five vital, basic material elements of nature and everything in the world is created by the motions among and differences of these five basic material elements and there is a dynamically balanced state through these relationships (Zimi Ma, 2014).

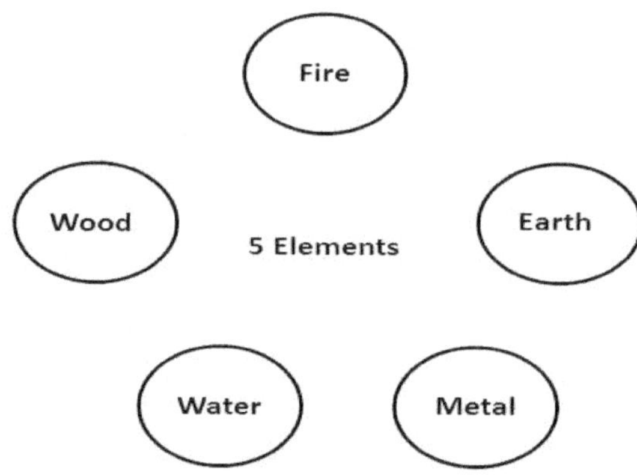

The Eight trigrams, also known as Bagua or Pa Kua are eight symbols derived from the yin and yang. Each symbol consists of three lines and each line either "broken" or "unbroken", that represent the fundamental principles of reality and a range of eight inter-related concepts (Wilhelm, 1967) (Wikipedia, Bagua, 2018).

Taoism or Daoism is considered by some people as a religion or philosophical tradition of Chinese origin which highlights living in harmony with the Tao (Chinese: 道; pinyin: Dào; "the Way"). Taoism contrasts from Confucianism by not emphasizing rigid rituals and social order (Pollard, Rosenberg, Tignor, Clifford, & Robert, 2011). The practice of Taoism varies according to the school, but overall emphasizes the three Treasures: 慈 "compassion", 儉 "frugality", and 不敢為天下先 "humility"; wu wei (action without intention), "naturalness", simplicity and spontaneity (Creel, 1970).

The Yin and Yang symbol or "double fish" is the symbol of the Chinese philosophy. The symbol means the duality of all things (Christensen, 2016). The idea is that opposite or contradictory forces may in fact be complementary, inter-connected and essential in every aspect of life. Examples of duality are: male and female, dark and light, fire and water, expanding and contracting and hard and soft. The dots in the symbols seem to refer that nothing is not only yin or yang or everything has yin and yang (Christensen, 2016)

The Tai Chi is inspired by the Neo-Confucianism (Christensen, 2016). Confucianism was founded by a Chinese philosopher, Master Kong (Confucius,

551-479 B.C.E.). It was based on the harmonious relationship between people in society, proper behaviour and a compassionate attitude towards others.

Confucianism is frequently referred to as a moral, ethical and a political system of thought or sometimes as a "religion philosophy". Martin Heidegger, German philosopher, and other modern and post-modern thinkers criticize the humanist tradition of thinking and suggest a return to the "mystical" and transcendent form of religion. In this context, Confucianism is viewed as human-centered systems of ethics, and morals (Was Confucianism a Religion or Philosophy? , 2018).

Confucians considered that Tai Chi is the Ultimate, an integrated energy of Yin and Yang which can be transformed into various forms. The ultimate source of all energy and knowledge is called Tao, which is the fundamental idea in most Chinese philosophical schools. Tao is related to how it works in the world, and how human beings relate to it. (Confucianism- Confucian Worldview, 2018) (What is Tao?, 2018).

In Summary, Confucianism and Taoism can be considered a philosophy or religion. It depends on the interpretation of what is considered a religion in our actual context. It is important to clarify that Tai Chi or others types of exercise like Yoga have their roots from different schools of thoughts, and they should not be considered as a religion. These exercises have been practiced by many people from different religions or traditions in different contexts.

3 CHAPTER
TAI CHI STYLES

"The journey of a thousand miles begins with one step."
Lao Tzu

The oldest styles of Tai Chi are: Chen, Yang and Wu. The main schools of Tai Chi are: Chen, Yang and Wu and most recently Sun style has increased in popularity. Most of the Tai Chi styles originated from at least one of the five traditional schools: Chen, Yang, Wu (Hao), Wu and Sun with their historical origins to Chen Village (Christensen, 2016).

Chen Style

The Chen family-style is the oldest form of Tai chi and is characterized by Silk reeling (a set of internal movement principles expressed in traditional styles of Tai Chi), alternating fast/slow motion and bursts of power (Guang Yi, 2003). Chen style was created in the seventeenth century by Chen Wangting, a royal guard who moved to retire to Chenjiagou Village. He belonged to the ninth generation of the Chen Clan and moved to the village because of the changes in the political context at the end of the Ming Dynasty and beginning of the Qing Dynasty. He included five routines of Tai Chi Chuan, 108 form Long Fist and a more rigorous routine known as Cannon Fist (Davidine Sim, 2002) (Chen-style t'ai chi ch'uan, 2018). Chen added principles of Yin and Yang philosophy, Daoyin (exercises practiced by Taoists) and Tui na (form of Chinese manipulative therapy used in conjunction with acupuncture, moxibustion, fire cupping, Chinese herbalism, Tai Chi and Qigong), theory of meridian, Chinese medical theory of energy and the boxing theories from sixteen different martial art styles (Chen-style t'ai chi ch'uan, 2018).

There are 16 essential principles for Chen style Tai Chi Chuan (Burr, 1999) (Chen-style t'ai chi ch'uan, 2018):

1) Keeping the head upright
2) Keeping the body straight
3) Drop the shoulders and sink the elbow
4) The chest curve inwards and the waist pressed forward
5) Sink the energy to the Dan Tian
6) Breath naturally
7) Relax the hip and keep the knees bent
8) The crotch is arch shaped
9) Keep the mind pure and clear
10) The top and bottom works together.

11) Adjust hardness and softness
12) Alternate fast and slow
13) The external shape is curved
14) The internal energy travels a spiral path
15) The body leads the hand
16) The waist is an axis

Yang Style

Yang Tai Chi is the most popular style which originated during the 19th century and is the most widely practised style in the world. The creator of Yang style was Yang Fu Kui, also known as Yang Lu Chan and as a young boy, Lu Chan studied Shaolin boxing skills. He was born in the Hebei province and studied in the Chen Clan which introduced it in Beijing.

Lots of resources purport that Yang Lu Chan was a servant in the Chen family and in the evening, he would secretly watch the Chen family practice their Tai Chi. However, one day the Chen family discovered that he was spying on them; the family could have very easily killed him, but upon discovering his talent for tai chi, they took him on as an "outdoor" student. Later on he developed his own style (Yang style) and became well-known when he was hired by the Chinese Imperial family to teach Tai Chi to the elite Palace Battalion of the Imperial Guards in 1850. He remained in this position until his death. Yang Style Tai Chi Chuan is typically done with slow, steady movements, extended and graceful, carefully structured, gentle and flowing movements, while still maintaining the martial arts aspects (Yang-style t'ai chi ch'uan, 2018).

Wu (Hao) Style

Wu (Hao) Style was created by Wu Yu-Xiang who studied both the Yang and Chen style and in the late 1800s he developed his own Wu Style. He was from a wealthy and influential family who financially supported him in his journey to learn Tai Chi with Chen Chang-Xiang. Yang transferred the knowledge to Wu because of the financial support after he returned from his Tai Chi studies. However, after Yang returned the third time, he could not teach Wu because he had promised his teacher he would not teach to other people. Then, in order to learn Tai Chi, Wu went to Chen Village. By that time, Chen Chang-Xiang was too old and referred him to a friend Chen Qing-Ping. Wu's older brother provided a book about Tai Chi classics to him and from that book together with his experience and practice, he developed the basis for Wu style Tai Chi. The

Wu style emphasises more internal requirements and has well-documented principles and its instruction is established on these theories.

Wu Style

The Wu Style is the second most popular form of Tai Chi in the world, after the Yang style (Yip Y. L., Autumn 2002). It is based on the small circle (Xiao Jia) form of Yang Tai Chi. Students also have more emphasis on the internal turning of the Dan Tian. The creator of this style was Wu Quanyou who was a student of Yang Lu Chan's son, Yang Banhou. Wu Quanyou was a military officer cadet of Manchu ancestry in the Yellow Banner camp in Beijing and also a hereditary officer of the Imperial Guards Brigade.

The smaller and restricted movements of the Wu Form have its origin in the restrictive clothes of the Imperial Court and it seems to be the reason why the movements of the original Yang Style were modified. He taught several students and his modifications to the art more evidently differentiate Wu style from Yang style (Philip-Simpson, June, 1995) (Wikipedia, Wu-style t'ai chi ch'uan, 2018).

Sun Style

Sun Lu-tang was the creator of the Tai Chi Sun Style. Before studying Tai Chi he was an expert in internal martial arts styles (xingyiquan and baguazhang). Sun learned first the Wu (Hao) style Tai Chi from Hao Weizhen (Li Yishe's chief disciple) (Wile, 1995). The Sun style has influence of xingyiquan, baguazhang and Wu (Hao) style. One of the similarities of the Sun style and Wu (Hao) style is the footwork. In both styles, when one foot advances and retreats, the other foot follows. The Sun style has higher stance, small circular movements with the hand and less kicking and punching (Yip L. , April, 1998).

4 CHAPTER

FUNDAMENTAL PRINCIPLES IN TAI CHI

"The journey of a thousand miles begins with one step."
Lao Tzu

There are some specific requirements for the practice of Tai Chi and it will differ according to the Tai Chi style that you are practicing.

The Tai Chi principles have some similarities with the pillars or fundamentals of Pilates exercises such as: breathing, concentration and flow. However, Tai Chi's "forms" or "postures" are more defined and emphasized than in Pilates exercises. The flow in Tai Chi is more similar to choreography or a dance in slow motion. That it is why Tai Chi is called the art of Tai Chi by some practitioners because in fact, it is also one form of art where the body moves with slow motions similar to a dance in the clouds. There are eight main fundamentals of Tai Chi as described below.

1) **Breathing**
2) **Balance**
3) **Concentration**
4) **Earthing (grounded)**
5) **Flow**
6) **Posture**
7) **Visualization (kinesthesia)**
8) **Weight transfer**

1. Breathing

Proper breathing is one of the fundamental principles of Tai Chi independent of the style you are practicing. Breathing is a physiological function that plays a vital role in removing carbon dioxide and supplying oxygen via blood circulation. Several researchers have already confirmed that a normal breathing pattern while performing exercise is essential for the success of rehabilitation programs and exercise effectiveness. Although the emphasis in breathing properly during exercises is already incorporated into many exercise practices such as yoga, Tai Chi, aikido, karate, capoeira, Pilates, dance, swimming and weightlifting, the recognition of the benefits of the actual breathing techniques has recently been growing in both Eastern and Western countries.

Tongue rest position:

This oral/tongue rest position is based on the principles of the Dan Tian breathing technique and it is also aligned with the recommendations of speech

pathologists and dentists/orofacial specialists. (K Rajeshwari, 2017)
- The lips should rest gently together.
- The teeth should be apart.
- The tongue-tip resting softly against the alveolar ridge, or back of the anterior top teeth, in a crescent shape -against the area of tissue which is located behind your upper front teeth. The tongue tip must rest on the incisive papilla, but the dorsum of the tongue should rest on the palate.
- The balance between the forces of orofacial muscles is essential in preserving good structural integrity. If the tongue rests on the palate, it will generate an outward force on the maxillary arch. This force is balanced by the inward forces of the buccinator muscles and the lips.
- The rest of the tongue, posterior to the tip, falls down and away from the palate.

Dan Tian breathing (dāntián,丹田)

This breathing method is based on the Taoism, which represents a school of thought that developed over a period of 200-300 years. It is a philosophical system developed by Lao-tzu and Chuang-tzu encouraging a simple life with harmony and non interference with the path (way) of natural events. Taoists believe that the universe is an abundant conduit of energy. This energy is known as Dan, or elixir. Taoists believe that energy exists in the universe and in people as well. This breathing method is based on traditional Qigong and improves qi power and enhances internal energy. It can be merged into all Qigong and Tai Chi movements. Doing these breathing exercises regularly leads to many health benefits: decreased blood pressure, slowing of heart rate, faster elimination of toxins, improved levels of circulating oxygen, reduced fatigue with exercise, reduced stress, and conditions such as post-traumatic stress, and depression and anxiety; and can also improve deep, core abdominal and pelvic floor muscle function. In Qigong terms, it signifies having energy in the center of the body. The center is called Dan Tian, which means "elixir field", "sea of qi", or simply "energy center". It is a place to store energy. Correct breathing is an essential part of any exercise program, including Tai Chi. Each time when you inhale, you are storing energy. When you exhale, you are delivering energy or power. The Dan Tian breathing exercise is described in the exercises section of this book.

2. Balance

Tai Chi is based on a System of Balance which is defined here as "a set of different theories and practices (Western and Eastern), interconnected to form a complex whole of balance between mind and body, body planes and postural stability and control"(Veras & Eagle Aalders, 2018).

There are different health theories and approaches in Western and Eastern countries. While Western medicine is an evidence-based science, Eastern medicine is based on the theory that an energy, called qi, circulates through channels called meridians. Western medicine defines health as "A state of complete physical, mental, and social well-being, and not merely the absence of disease or infirmity." (WHO, Constitution of WHO: principles, 2018). In contrast, Eastern medicine believes that health is a balanced state versus disease as an unbalanced state. Western science has its roots in the philosophy of Ancient Greece and the Renaissance and hypothetical deduction. Eastern medicine was developed in China more than 2000 years ago based on the Yin and Yang theory and Five Phases theory (wood, fire, earth, metal and water) and an inductive method. The Western approach is grounded on the modern philosophy of Descartes where the disease is studied and treated based on the location of his body part instead of the whole body and mind connected (Accad, 2016). For the Eastern countries, the individual is viewed upon as a small universe. The anatomical parts of the body and the physiological functions of the body are interconnected with one another and influenced by the outside environment, the large universe. Within this theory the health is a state of balance between the continuing changes on the physiological process and the environment conditions. Diseases will occur only if this balance is disturbed (Julia J. Tsuei, 1978). The System of Balance described here recognizes these theories, philosophies and approaches and aims to integrate them into Tai Chi for rehabilitation and wellness.

The body planes are imaginary lines (vertical or horizontal) drawn through an upright body to describe the location of structures or the direction of movements. There are three main planes used in anatomy: the sagittal plane, the coronal plane, and the transverse plane. The sagittal plane or median plane is a plane parallel to the sagittal suture, perpendicular to the ground and divides the body into left and right. The coronal plane or frontal plane (vertical) divides the body into dorsal and ventral (back and front, or posterior and anterior) portions. The transverse plane or axial plane (lateral, horizontal) is parallel to the ground and divides the body into cranial and caudal (head and tail) portions (Wikipedia, Anatomical plane, 2018). The System of Balance aims to integrate upper and lower body, left and right sides and anterior and posterior body anatomical planes.

Postural stability and control refers to the individual's ability to maintain their line of gravity within their Base of Support (BOS) (Shumway-Cook A, 2007). Balance is essential for many functional activities of daily life such as mobility and fall prevention. Balance impairment can occur after an injury as well as with ageing; nearly 30% of older adults over 65 experience one or more falls every year and up to 75% of people aged 70 years or older, leading to hospitalization and death (Kathryn M. Sibley, 2011) (Nima Toosizadeh, 2018). In the human body, the balance system and balance control is very complex and involves many different underlying systems such as the Somatosensory/Proprioceptive System, Vestibular System and Visual System. The Somatosensory/Proprioceptive System is part of the sensory nervous system and is made of sensory neurons and pathways that respond to variations at the surface or inside the body. Sensory receptors are found all over the body including the skin, epithelial tissues, internal organs, musculoskeletal system and cardiovascular system. The sensory nervous system is responsible for providing information about the position of different parts of the body with respect to one another, pain, proprioception, temperature and touch. Proprioception is essential for maintaining posture and balance because the somatosensory proprioceptive cues are combined with vestibular proprioceptive cues and visual cues to control motor responses to variations in head and body position. (Toosizadeh, Ehsani, Miramonte, & and Mohler, 2018) (Dougherty, 2018).

The Visual System is part of the central nervous system and composed of six extra-ocular muscles and millions of light-sensitive sensors, called rod and cone receptors, which make up the retina of the eye and provides organisms the ability to process visual detail, as well as enabling the formation of numerous non-image photo response functions (ScienceDirect, 2018). Visual function unavoidably deteriorates with age, and the deterioration of visual function affects the balance and in turn increases fall risk (Nafisa Saftari, 2018).

The Vestibular System is an integral part of the labyrinth that lies in the otic capsule in the petrous portion of the temporal bone [the "inner ear"]. It is responsible for noticing the position and motion of the head, mainly angular motions such as rotation. This system stabilizes the eyes when the head is moving and adjusting in body position (Swenson, 2018). Vestibular dysfunction is present in around one-third of all people over 40 years old and frequently results in disturbed standing balance control and increased risk of falling (Agrawal Y, 2009).

The Vestibular System, in collaboration with the Visual System and the Somatosensory System estimate the body lean angle with respect to the environment during standing balance control (Peterka, 2001). There is a growing body of evidence that Tai Chi may be an important complementary treatment for vestibular disorders. A study comparing Tai Chi with vestibular rehabilitation intervention demonstrated that Tai Chi improved lower extremity motor control more than vestibular rehabilitation, producing better trunk control and a more vigorous gait (A McGibbon, et al., 2005). The System of

Balance in Tai Chi integrates and recognizes the important role of the Somatosensory/Proprioceptive System, Vestibular System and Visual System and the association with balance control.

3. Concentration

Tai Chi practice requires concentration, focus and mindfulness. The ability to practice the postures and name them demands attention, concentration and memory (Rainbow Tin Hung Ho, 2014). It also improves mental, intentional vigilance and executive control. When practicing Tai Chi, you need to be mindful of all parts of your body, your posture and your balance. Tai Chi requires a combination of mind and body; mental and physical activity work to bring the mind, body and spirit into harmony. It also contributes to generate energy movement and well-being.

4. Earthing (grounded)

Tai Chi is practiced in a standing position with feet on the ground; your body is connected with the earth. The goal is to create a deeper connection to the ground, both physically and mentally. Earthing and grounded are related to roots. In general, the term, "roots", is correlated with fundamentals, essentials, basics, causes, origins, etc.

One of the Five Elements, Phases or Forces is the Earth Element. The Earth Element is associated with mothers, nurturing, stability, patience, rootedness, inwardness, centering, practicality, late summer, yellow, planet Saturn, spleen, stomach, mouth, thoughtfulness, muscles, empathy, responsibility, long-term planning and the Yellow Dragon. Earth is a balance of both yin and yang and brings both the feminine and masculine together.

The modern life has disconnected us to the earth - to be "grounded". Being ungrounded is a global epidemic deeply embedded in people and it has contributed to many mobility problems, musculoskeletal injuries and mental health problems. When we are not connected to the ground, we are frequently using cars for transportation instead of active transportation such as walking or we are in a seated position at a desk for work or just browsing social media websites for recreation. In fact, research suggests that this "disconnect" may be a main contributor to physiological dysfunction.

Emerging evidence shows that contact with the Earth (being outside barefoot or indoors connected to grounded conductive systems) is a very effective environmental strategy to prevent chronic stress, inflammation, pain, poor sleep, nerve dysfunction, disturbed heart rate variability, hypercoagulable blood, and cardiovascular disease (Gaétan Chevalier, Oschman, Sokal, & Sokal, 2012). A recent study about reducing sitting time in free-living conditions demonstrated that replacing sitting with standing and self-perceived light walking is an effective strategy to improve insulin sensitivity, circulating lipids, diastolic blood pressure, to improve cardio-metabolic risk factors in overweight and obese participants (Duvivier, et al., 2017). Another study about the health implications of reconnecting the human body to the earth's surface electrons, showed that grounding reduces or even prevents the cardinal signs of inflammation following injury such as redness, heat, pain, swelling, and loss of function. Electrically conductive contact of the human body with the earth produces immune responses, wound healing, prevention and treatment of chronic inflammatory and autoimmune diseases (Oschman, Chevalier, & Brown, 2015). Grounding also has effect on mood. A study was conducted to assess if Earthing improves mood in adult participants. The results demonstrated that pleasant and positive moods statistically significantly improved among grounded participants. The author concluded that the Earth improved mood more than expected by relaxation alone (Chevalier, 2015).

The practice of Tai Chi contributes to the reconnection with the Earth's electrons and may contribute to the promotion of intriguing physiological benefits and well-being. Tai Chi also maximizes the way in which your body draws energy from the earth into the body systems.

5. Flow

Practicing Tai Chi is described by many experts as being like a "moving meditation". The goal of Tai Chi is to facilitate the body's pathways and get the fluids flowing freely through the body. The optimal energy can be used to heal or used as self-defense.

One of the Tai Chi principles described by Paul Cavel, author and Tai Chi teacher, is about moving like a puppet or string, where the head is suspended as if connected to the sky, but he affirms that the head does not lift up the body. Instead, the spine does at C7-T1. He describes that the arms are elevated by the wrists or fingers, facilitating the hands to be empty, open and not heavy. Elbows and shoulders move downwards with the flow of the gravity. The knee drives the lift of the leg, letting the foot to keep the position in a relaxed posture (Carvel, 2017).

6. Posture

Dynamic and static body postures are a crucial characteristic of Tai Chi. Tai Chi is a fabulous exercise to create awareness of a good posture and body alignment. During Tai Chi practice, you need to pay attention from the beginning to the end of the postures or movements. The good posture is highlighted in traditional Tai Chi books, for example:

"The postures should be without defect, without hollows or projections from the proper alignment"; "Every joint in your body must be strung together. This allows qi to pass smoothly through your body and benefits both form and application", (Lo et al., 1979) (Osypiuk, Thompson, & and Wayne, 2018) and "Keep the tailbone (coccyx) centrally aligned and straight so the spirit of vitality (shen) penetrates up to the crown of the head. Then, with the head feeling as if suspended from above, the entire body will be light and agile" (Lo et al., 1979) (Osypiuk, Thompson, & and Wayne, 2018).

The performance of the postures or movements in Tai Chi is in consonance with the body mind relationship. "These forms are not the means of obtaining a right state of mind. To take this posture is itself to have the right state of mind" (Suzuki, 1970).

Some authors have introduced and explored the hypothesis that body postures in Tai Chi might be one biological element contributing to improvements in psychological well-being. The authors had developed an evolutionary framework for understanding the interdependence of posture and emotion. They mentioned that Charles Darwin has already well-described his observation of physical expressions of emotion and movements associated with specific states of mind (Osypiuk, Thompson, & and Wayne, 2018). According to the authors, Darwin identified depression and grief emotions or states of mind related to a contracted, flaccid, downwardly sinking posture. Differently, cheerfulness is associated with erect, upright, open posture of high spirits (Osypiuk, Thompson, & and Wayne, 2018).

Another study about the differences and similarities in postural alterations caused by sadness and depression investigated if there is an association between sadness, depression and the posture represented by the angle of Tales, head inclination, shoulder inclination, and forward head and shoulder protrusion. The study participants were women, aged between 20 and 30 years, with normal body mass indices and not having a diagnosis of neurological, psychiatric, or musculoskeletal disorders. The results of the study demonstrated that there is an association between posture and depression. Inclination of the shoulders was associated with current sadness ($p = 0.03$; $r = 0.443$) and usual sadness ($p = 0.04$; $r = 0.401$). In addition to that, usual sadness was also associated with protrusion of the shoulder ($p = 0.05$; $r = 0.492$). The authors of this study concluded and recommend that postural assessment and treatment may contribute in diagnosing and treating depression (Rosario, Bezerra-Diógenes, Mattei, & Leite, 2014).

The posture is an important principal of Tai Chi not only from the physical aspect, but also from the physiological aspects providing both physical and psychological benefits. From the Eastern perspective, a good posture and body alignment provides an optimal pathway for the flow of qi in the body.

7. Visualization (kinesthesia)

Kinesthetic feedback occurs when you practice Tai Chi postures or movements. Kinesthesia or kinæsthesia (kinesthetic sense) is defined as sensation and awareness of the position and movement of the parts of the body. Kinesthesia is an important component in muscle memory and eye-hand co-ordination, and training can improve this sense.

Many Tai Chi practitioners refer to a "weird sensation" that occurs when practicing Tai Chi. In fact, when you practice Tai Chi in your backyard, park or other places, your body creates "memory" of your moves in that environment. When you try to practice in different places or even in the same room, but in a different location of the room, sometimes you may struggle to perform the movements and postures.

There is a description that if you use the same clothes, it may help you to bring this memory back. A Tai Chi expert has already described that he was able to remember the postures because of the sensation of the clothes moving on his body. He has an interesting description: "sleeves dragging and tightening on my arms at certain points and my shirt instructed me where to go based on what constriction or freeness I was anticipating. " (Tai Chi Clothing, 2018).

Cognitive neuroscience recognizes that kinesthetic awareness is part of many movement-based introspective practices such as Tai Chi, Yoga and Qigong and they are based on the concepts of embodiment, movement and contemplation (Schmalzl, Crane-Godreau, & and Payne, 2014). Embodiment includes a complex interaction of brain, body and environment, and integration of interoceptive, proprioceptive, vestibular, kinesthetic, tactile, and spatial information (Haselager, Broens, & Gonzalez, 2012).

The concept of "movement-based" includes very delicate and imagined, movement. The idea of imaginary movement is supported by the concepts of neural mechanisms underlying motor control and motor imagery where each performance of an overt movement controlled by the primary motor cortex is preceded by activations in premotor cortex (one of the principal brain areas involved in motor function) and supplementary motor areas (Haselager, Broens, & Gonzalez, 2012). The role of the primary motor cortex is to generate neural impulses that control the execution of movement. The supplementary motor area is responsible for assisting with the planning of complex movements and in co-ordinating two-handed movements.

Neurophenomenology is the theoretical approach that is fundamental to the investigation of contemplative and meditative practices such as Tai Chi, Yoga and Qigong. This approach was developed for systematizing the use of first-person methods and introspective phenomenological reports in the study of subjective conscious experience. It also associates the information collected through those techniques to complex dynamical systems analysis of brain activity (Haselager, Broens, & Gonzalez, 2012).

First-person methods (phenomenological, meditative or psychotherapeutic) increase an individual's sensitivity and attention to the quality of their experience while they practice these methods. These experiences are described in phenomenology as "epoché" and consists of three phases: 1) Suspension of habitual thoughts, 2) Redirection of attention to the experience itself, and 3) Receptivity to whatever arises from it (Depraz, Varela, Vermersch, & P., 2000) (Husserl, 2012) (Haselager, Broens, & Gonzalez, 2012).

Several studies have indicated that Kinesthesia is an effective approach to add to a rehabilitation program. A study was conducted with participants age 50 years or older to determine the efficacy of a home-based kinesthesia, balance and agility exercise program to improve symptoms of knee osteoarthritis. Results indicate that these exercises seem effective in reducing symptoms and improving the quality of life of people with knee osteoarthritis (Rogers, Tamulevicius, Semple, & Krkeljas, 2012). Another study about the effect of a kinesthetic illusion in patients who had stroke indicated that this approach can acutely affect motor function positively in patients with stroke. Kinesthetic illusion is believed to induce a feeling as if a person's own body is moving during sensory input, despite the fact that the body is in a resting state (Kaneko, Inada, Matsuda, Koyama, & Shibata, 2015).

Another study has also investigated the role of kinesthesia in mental health and pain management. The study investigated the influence of trait anxiety and illusory kinesthesia on pain threshold. The results of the study demonstrated that illusory kinesthesia has the effect of increasing the pain threshold (Ryota, Michihiro, & Tomoya, 2017). Tai Chi exercises also affect kinesthesia of the lower limb joints of older adult women. Results showed that the 24 week Tai Chi intervention significantly improved the kinesthesia of the ankle dorsiflexion and knee flexion and extension (Cheng, Chang, Li, & Hong, 2017).

8. Weight Transfer

One of the most important principles of Tai Chi is weight transfer. This is probably the most complex and physically demanding skill required during Tai Chi movements. However, with practice and commitment, it becomes natural and over time, strengthens the legs. During practice of the postures or movements, weight shift assists with separating Yin and Yang and full and empty footwork.

Effects of Tai Chi on balance are well-described in the literature. The benefits of practicing weight transfer for improving balance is reported for people with neurological disease and also for the healthy population. A randomized, controlled trial study was conducted to determine whether a tailored tai chi program could improve postural control in patients with idiopathic Parkinson's disease. The authors concluded that Tai Chi was effective to reduce balance impairments, improve functional capacity and reduce falls in patients with mild to moderate Parkinson's disease (Li, et al., 2012). A study comparing static and dynamic balance in healthy elderly practitioners of Tai Chi versus ballroom dancing demonstrated that the Tai Chi group had faster walking speeds, shorter transfer times, and better postural balance in the final standing position during the performance of the Sit-to-Stand Test (Rahal, et al., 2015).

Another benefit of weight transfer in Tai Chi is the increase of bone density. Several systematic reviews have been published examining the protective effect of Tai Chi for people who are experiencing bone mineral density loss. A recent systematic review and meta-analysis of randomized controlled trials was conducted to determine the effects of practicing Tai Chi on attenuating bone mineral density loss. The study findings indicated that a long-term Tai Chi practice (around 24 weeks) may be an effective intervention to attenuate bone density loss in several areas of the body such as lumbar spine, proximal femur neck and trochanter, especially in perimenopausal and postmenopausal women, older adults, breast cancer survivors, women with osteoarthritis (Zou, et al., 2017).

5 CHAPTER
CLOTHES AND SHOES IN TAI CHI

"Wherever you go, go with all your heart."
Confucius

1) Clothes

Although you can find many people using uniforms for special occasions, the basic premise for practicing Tai Chi is using conformable clothes. Different from Yoga, Pilates or other types of exercises, the best option for Tai Chi clothes includes the ones that are not tight, are soft, light, made from fabrics such as cotton, linen, or silk, and supple enough to facilitate the postures. Traditional Chinese martial arts practitioners promote silk and linen for pants as a good choice because linen is thermo-regulating, strong and durable. There is no restriction for colors, unless there is a specific color of some schools. To simplify, many schools adhere to a printed T-shirt as the school uniform and loose pants. However, the most important component for practicing Tai Chi is really a state of mind, where you are mindful of your practice. The clothes will help you only if your mind is already engaged into the practice to guide your moves with flow and precision. Tai Chi is known to be a meditation in movement; therefore your mind should be focused on your moves and not distracted (Teahupoo, 2018). The underlying concept of wearing this type of clothing is because according to the Tai Chi philosophy, the qi is moving inside and outside of the body and needs to move freely.

Shoes

There is not a mandated type of shoe for Tai Chi. Some people like to use sneakers; others prefer plain Tai Chi cotton shoes and there are some who have a preference for socks or even to go barefoot. The most important thing is to have shoes that allow your feet to move freely during your practice. You should avoid shoes that have high friction which can put strain on the knee if there is any drag.

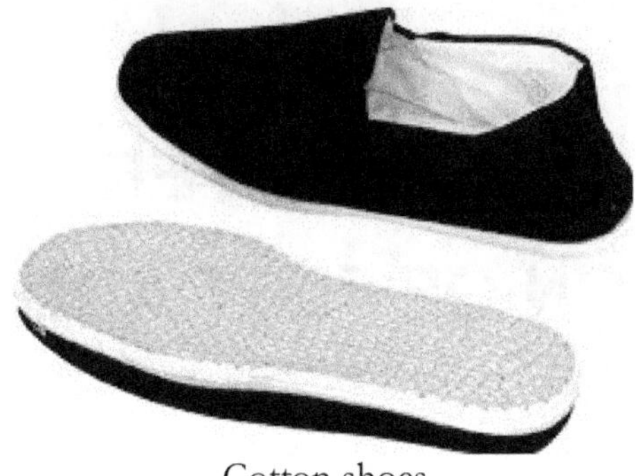

Cotton shoes

There is also some mixed information about whether to practice Tai Chi barefoot or not. Some reasons for practicing Tai Chi barefoot come from the philosophical principles of Tai Chi as well as new research in the practice of exercising barefoot. Based on the philosophical principle of Tai Chi, if you practice Tai Chi without shoes, it can provide you with the experience of being grounded – i.e. earthing. Barefoot practice also stimulates several acupuncture points on the soles of the feet and enhances the flow of energy during a Tai Chi practice.

From the scientific perspective, research in running barefoot or in minimalist shoes has recently gained popularity and attention of the scientific community. Several benefits have been discussed and described in the literature such as injury prevention, enhanced running efficiency, cognitive benefits and improved performance compared with running in shoes (Perkins, Hanney, & Rothschild, 2014). A study that investigated the cognitive benefit found that working memory can be improved after at least 16 minutes of barefoot running if the individual had emphasised attention on the ground (Alloway, Alloway, Magyari, & Floyd, 2016). Overall, there is a lack of high-quality evidence on the benefits and no definitive conclusions can be made at this time regarding the potential risks and benefits of running barefoot or in minimalist shoes (Perkins, Hanney, & Rothschild, 2014). Remember that people who have diabetes or plantar fasciitis will need to use good shoes to avoid injury and/or infection.

6 CHAPTER
POSITION OF FEET AND HANDS

> *"Simplicity, patience, compassion.*
> *These three are your greatest treasures.*
> *Simple in actions and thoughts, you return to the source of being.*
> *Patient with both friends and enemies,*
> *you accord with the way things are.*
> *Compassionate toward yourself,*
> *you reconcile all beings in the world."*
>
> *— Lao Tzu, Tao Te Ching*

Foot

The foot work is the most important part of Tai Chi because good footwork will provide balance and control which is absolutely fundamental when practicing Tai Chi. If the footwork is not performed properly, you will have a hard time performing the next form or posture correctly. The three crucial characteristics of good footwork are:

1) Safe transfer (transfer your weight to one foot before you attempt to lift your other foot);

2) Place your foot securely on the ground before you transfer your weight to it (to prevent you from losing your balance and be able to adjust your stance) and

3) Use only your legs to guide the transfer of your weight (King, 2018). These elements are important to contribute to improved balance, flexibility and reducing the risk of fall. Tai Chi also can contribute to improved awareness of the body's position by concentrating on the proper placement of the foot, maintaining a good posture, and moving the body into different postures (Liu, 2010). For a correct footwork you should pay attention to your balance, stability and awareness of your movements.

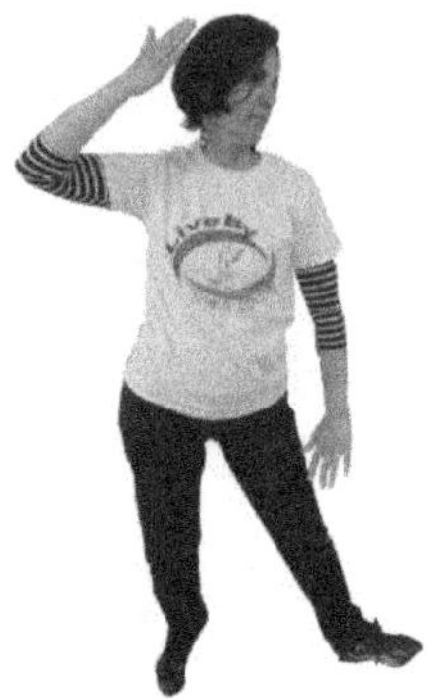

Types of Footwork in Tai Chi

"Water is fluid, soft and yielding. But water will wear away rock, which is rigid and cannot yield. As a rule, whatever is fluid, soft and yielding will overcome whatever is rigid and hard. This is another paradox: what is soft is strong."
Lao-Tzu

Many Tai Chi experts describe footwork for Tai Chi; others prefer to call it as "Tai Chi Stance". In fact, both terms are appropriate since the positions of the feet are critical for the stance adopted in the postures. For didactic proposes, it is described here as footwork used for Tai Chi stances.

1) Bow Stance

Bow stance is also called "arrow step" or arched step". This stance is the foundation of many Tai Chi movements and is the most frequently utilized stance in Yang style Tai Chi. To perform the Bow stance you should follow the steps:
1)   Standing with both feet parallel and about hip-width apart.
2)   Turn your right foot out slightly around 45 degrees by turning on your heel to point your toes outward.
3)   Transfer approximately 60 to 70% of your weight onto your front leg, and bend your knee. Your stance will looks like a lunge.
4)   Align your hips so that they are also facing forward, but remember to respect the limits of your hip flexibility.
5)   Keep your front knee aligned with the toes of the front foot.

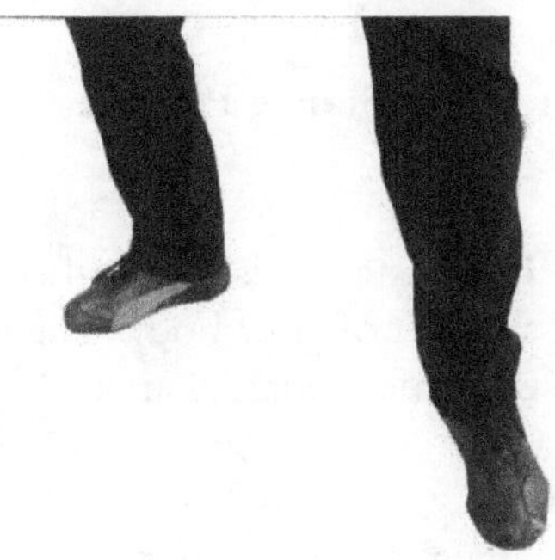

Bow stance

2)   Empty Step

The "empty" step is the perfect example of balance in Tai Chi and carries the philosophical concept of yin and yang. When you have one foot in "empty" step the other foot will carry your weight. Some examples where you are going to use this footwork is during your performance of the movements of "Play the lute/pipa" or "play the guitar" or also "white crane" movement. Usually, the majority of the weight is on one leg while the other leg is just resting on the floor, usually on the heel.

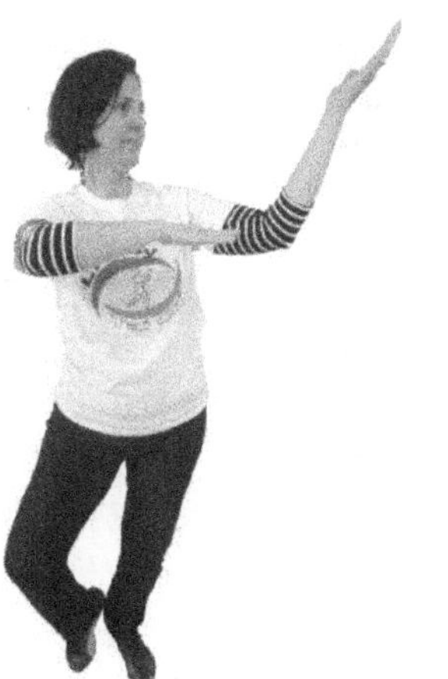 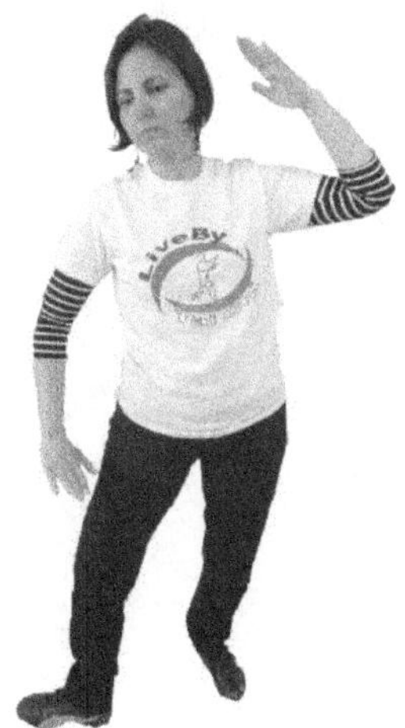

2) Horse Foot in Horse Stance Posture

The footwork for horse stance is performed with your feet flat on the ground giving you full support of your body. The position assumed is similar to riding a horse and is used in many martial arts.

How to perform it:

1) You stand up straight, and then put your legs apart and feet facing forward.

2) Bend your knees and lower the trunk and upper body as if you were sitting on horse for a ride (make sure that your knees are not forward or outward over the toes).

3) Feel your upper body resting on your hips and legs. This posture was created for superior stability of the body.

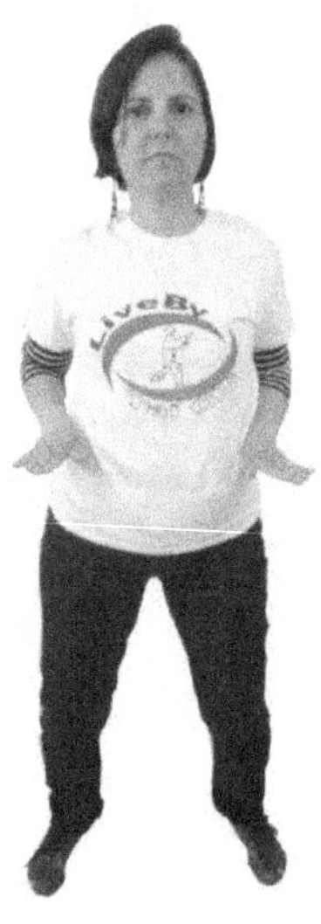

7 CHAPTER
TYPES OF HAND POSITIONS IN TAI CHI

"Knowing others is intelligence;
knowing yourself is true wisdom.
Mastering others is strength;
mastering yourself is true power."
— Lao Tzu, Tao Te Ching

Like the feet, there are different hand positions for the dynamic postures in Tai Chi. Many Tai Chi postures imitate animal postures and the most common of them are described below:

Hooked Hands

The hook hand is a hand with your wrist bent, fingers and thumb pressed together and arched downward in the form of a claw, similar to pinching salt with your fingers. The hook hand posture is also a technique of training the wrist and improving finger power. This hand posture is used for Single Whip in the Tai Chi Yang style.

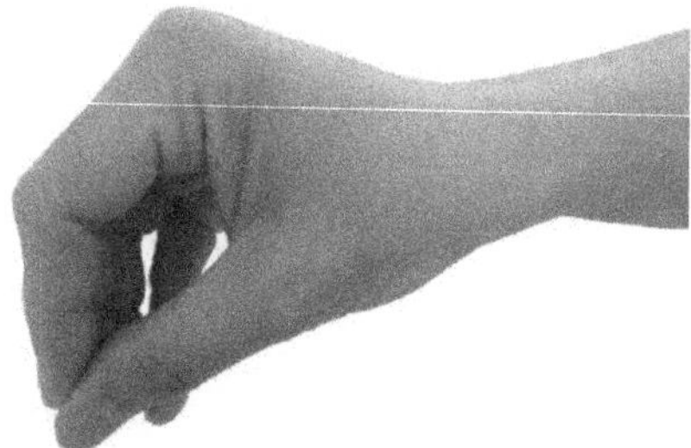

Hooked hands

Tiger Paw

Start with your fingers straight, slowly curl them back, and hold this position. The hands imitate the shape and movement of a tiger and its attitude of strength and ferocity.

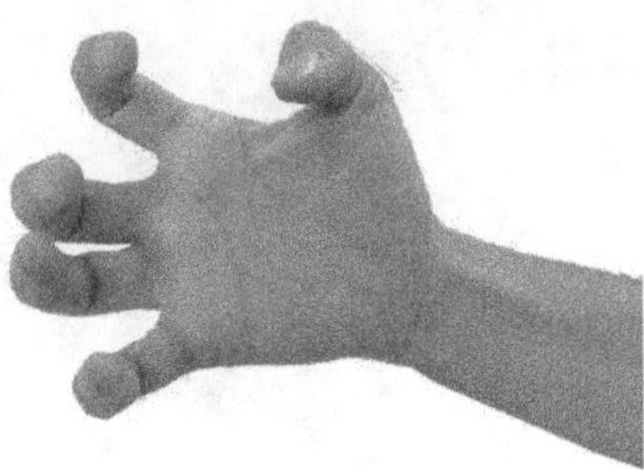

Bear Hands

Hands more relaxed with wrist gently bent.

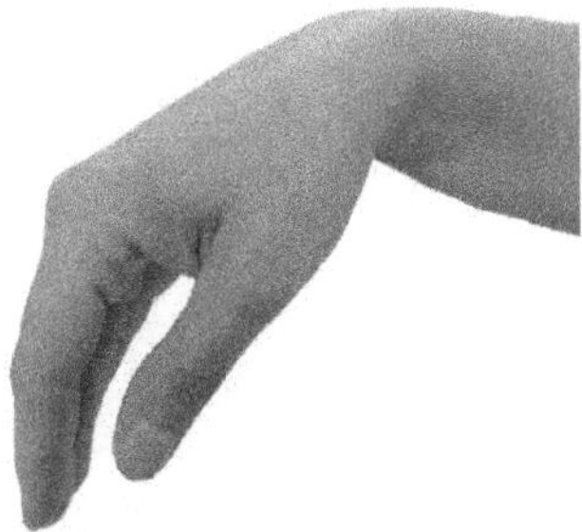

Deer Hands

You start by making a "letter C" with your thumb and second finger. Then the second finger rests on top of the third finger. The 4th and 5th fingers are apart from each other as well as from the other fingers.

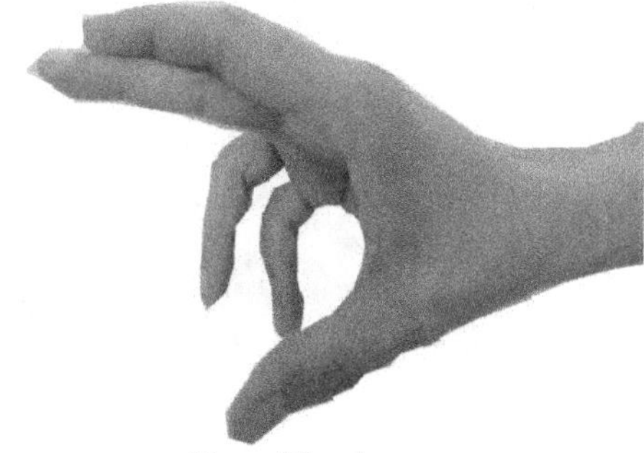

Deer Hands

8 CHAPTER

WHY ADD TAI CHI IN YOUR REHABILITATION PROGRAM?

"When you are content to be simply yourself and don't compare or compete, everyone will respect you."

— *Lao Tzu, Tao Te Ching*

The most important component of a rehabilitation program is the exercise. The utilization of different exercise styles such as Pilates and yoga has been significantly growing in the rehabilitation field. Tai Chi exercises are a fun way to increase the effectiveness of patients' outcomes by increasing motivation for performing the exercises in a supervised clinical environment or for a home exercise program. Some benefits to add Tai Chi in your rehabilitation program are:

- To improve posture

- To increase motor control function

- To empower people to wellness

- To improve mental health status

- Can be easily and quickly integrated into clinical practice

- Improve respiratory function

- Improve exercise adherence

- Improve sleep and quality of life

- Increase flexibility

- Reduce blood pressure

- Reduce fear and risk of falls

- Improve balance

- Improve cognition

9 CHAPTER

TAI CHI FOR CHRONIC PAIN AND REHABILITATION IS EVIDENCE-BASED

Several studies have demonstrated the effectiveness of Tai Chi for chronic pain. Tai Chi exercises are usually recommended to manage chronic pain from osteoarthritis, rheumatoid arthritis, low back pain, neck pain, and fibromyalgia. (Lee, 2011) (Vitetta, 2005) (Wang, 2009). The exercises are performed with slow motions and weight shifting which can be beneficial for joint stability, flexibility and musculoskeletal strength (Wang, 2009).

A systematic review and meta analysis of studies with randomized controlled trials regarding Tai Chi for chronic pain conditions was conducted and it included 18 randomized controlled trials with participants who had chronic pain conditions (duration of more than 6 months). The result of the review showed that Tai Chi accomplished better improvements in ameliorating chronic pain compared to the control interventions (SMD, -0.65; 95% CI, -0.82 to -0.48; $P<0.001$) (Ling Jun Kong, 2016). The aggregated results indicated that Tai Chi significantly improved low back pain, rheumatoid arthritis, osteoporosis and fibromyalgia. Three studies included in this review tested the effects of Tai Chi for herpes zoster (post herpetic pain), rheumatoid arthritis, and stroke reported that Tai Chi exercise was more effective in reducing pain from herpes zoster when compared with health education (mean changes, 6.68 versus 3.79, $P< 0.05$)25) (Ling Jun Kong, 2016). Tai Chi also demonstrated reducing pain in patients who had stroke compared to physiotherapy treatment (mean changes, 5.55 versus 0.82, $P< 0.05$) (Ling Jun Kong, 2016).

Lan and colleagues also found that a 12-months Tai Chi training program could significantly increase participants' thoracolumbar flexibility (Lan C, 12-monts Tai Chi training in the elderly: its effect on health fitness, 1998) and a 6-months Tai Chi practice was effective in enhancing the strength of knee extensors (Lan C, Tai Chi Chuan to improve muscular strength and endurance in elderly individuals: a pilot study, 2000). A study demonstrated that after practicing Tai Chi, men had a 13.5% to 24.2% increase in isokinetic strength in concentric contractions, and a 15.1% to 23.8% increase in eccentric contractions (Jacobson BH, 1997).

Tai Chi for mental health and cognitive challenges

Since Tai Chi is a mindfulness exercise where a person needs to concentrate in the present moment and in the movements that are performed, Tai Chi helps to reduce chronic pain (Tsai, 2013). Tai Chi has been shown to be effective to reduce stress, anxiety and depression. A systematic review and meta-analysis were carried out on studies about the effects of tai chi on psychological well-being. The results of this study indicated that Tai Chi have beneficial effects for people with depression, anxiety or general stress. (Wang F, 2014). Another study demonstrated that Tai Chi was effective to lower summary depression scores, lower anxiety scores and lower sleep disturbances scores (Field T, 2013). It has also been reported in a study that Tai Chi exercises increases brain volume and enhances memory and thinking scores and it can be effective in combating dementia illnesses like Alzheimer's (James A. Mortimer, 2012).

Studies demonstrated that Tai Chi interventions reduce musculoskeletal pain, improve emotion, cognition, and physical function in individuals with posttraumatic stress disorder (Tsai PF1, 2017). Tai Chi has effects on cognitive functions and plasma biomarkers such as brain-derived neurotrophic factor (BDNF), tumour necrosis factor-α (TNF-α), and interleukin-10 (IL-10) in older adults with mild cognitive impairment. A study demonstrated that Tai Chi significantly improved memory and the mental switching component of executive function in older adults with a mild cognitive impairment, perhaps through an up-regulation of BDNF (Sungkarat S, 2018). According to another study, Tai Chi can significantly increase grey matter volume (GMV) in the insula, medial temporal lobe, and putamen after 12-weeks of exercise. It also has the potential for the prevention of memory deficits in older adults (Tao J, 2017).

Overall, Tai Chi improves well-being, mental concentration, breathing, and has positive physical and mental effects. These studies regarding the mental and physical benefits of Tai Chi indicated great potential for becoming widely integrated into the clinician's practice for prevention and rehabilitation of a number of physical and psychological conditions (Wang F, 2014).

Tai Chi for preventing falls in older adults

Falls are a major, costly, public health problem worldwide. According to the World Health Organization (WHO), globally, falls are the second leading cause of accidental or unintentional injury and deaths. The greatest number of fatal falls is among adults older than 65 years of age. Additionally, each year 37.3 million falls occur that are severe enough to require hospitalization or medical attention. The WHO emphasizes that preventative approaches should include education, training, creating safer environments, prioritizing fall-related research and effective policies to reduce risks (WHO, WHO Global Report on Falls Prevention in Older Age., 2018) (Scheffer AC, 2008) (Lomas-Vega R, 2017).

There is a growing interest in the effectiveness of Tai Chi for improving balance, co-ordination and prevention of falls in older adults. Tai Chi is an ancient physical activity in which several studies have demonstrated that Tai Chi is an effective, evidence-based exercise in prevention of falls through improving balance, flexibility, muscle strength, activities of daily living and a reduced fear of falling (4-8).

A systematic review and meta-analysis was conducted to assess the preventive effect of Tai Chi by updating the latest trial evidence. The study included sixteen studies with a total of 3539 participants. The results indicated that the chances of falling at least once was lower in the Tai Chi group when compared to the control group (RR 0.80, 90% CI 0.72 to 0.88); heterogeneity: p=0.1, 1=32%). Tai Chi significantly reduced the number of fallers (20%) and the rate of falls (31%). (Zhi-Guan Huang, 2017)here. Insert chapter ten text here.

10 CHAPTER
TAI CHI FOR USE IN REHABILITATION

"There is no mystique to Tai Chi Chuan. What is difficult is the perseverance. It took me ten years to discover my chi, but thirty years to learn how to use it. Once you see the benefit, you won't want to stop."
- Ma Yueh Liang

This chapter has exercises based on adapted Tai Chi for use in a rehabilitation or preventive, wellness program. The exercises were developed based on a level of complexity from low to moderate. However, you have to assess your population each time you prescribe the exercises in order to prevent injuries and take into account their baselines in flexibility and physical limitations.

Tai Chi Level I- Beginning

1.Breathing Exercises

1.1 Dan Tian breathing (dāntián,丹田)

This breathing method is based on Taoism, which represents a school of thought that developed over a period of 200-300 years. It is a philosophical system developed by Lao-tzu and Chuang-tzu encouraging a simple life with harmony and non interference with the path (way) of natural events. Taoists believe that the universe is an abundant conduit of energy. This energy is known as Dan, or elixir. Taoists believe that energy exists in the universe and in people as well. This breathing method is based on traditional Qigong and improves qi power and enhances internal energy. It can be merged into all Qigong and Tai Chi movements. Doing these breathing exercises regularly leads to many health benefits: decreased blood pressure, slowing of heart rate, faster elimination of toxins, improved levels of circulating oxygen, reduced fatigue with exercise, reduced stress, post-traumatic stress, and depression and anxiety; and also improved deep, core abdominal and pelvic floor muscle function. In Qi gong terms, it signifies having energy in the center of the body. The center is called Dan Tian, which means "elixir field", "sea of qi", or simply "energy center". It is a place to store energy. Correct breathing is an essential part of any exercise program, including for Tai Chi. Each time you inhale, you are storing energy. When you exhale, you are delivering energy or power.

Objective: Breathing exercises are recommended to activate the diaphragm muscle, pelvic floor muscles, expand the lungs, and induce the body's relaxation response. This technique allows your body to take in more oxygen and release more carbon dioxide.

Location of Dan Tian: It is located in your lower belly, and it is the natural center for your body's energy. It is two (or three) finger-breadths below the navel and two (or three) finger-breadths in.

How to perform

Step 1: You can perform this exercise sitting down in a chair, lying down or in a standing position. Close your eyes (if you feel comfortable), and let the breath gradually come and go as it will.

Step 2: As you begin to relax, slowly place the feeling aspect of your mind into your lower Dan Tian and leave it there.

Step 3: Breathe in slowly and deeply so that you feel your belly rise under your hand. You may also notice your lower rib cage move wide under your other hand. The focus is keeping the upper chest muscles relaxed and using the diaphragm to breathe. When you breathe in, expand your lower abdominal area and let your abdominal and pelvic floor muscles relax.

Step 4: Exhale slowly through your mouth and feel your lower belly contract.

For pelvic floor activation:

Exhale by letting the rib cage fall back to resting. You should feel a gentle rise and fall of your belly under your hand. As you exhale, gently contract the pelvic floor muscles and the lower abdomen.

Cueing for pelvic floor activation:

> **Females** - Visualize stopping urine flow ('squeezing'/close off the urethra), hold this while you 'squeeze'/close the anus (as if to stop flatulence/gas) and then, gently lift.

> **Males** - visualize gently drawing your testicles up and forward into your abdomen.

Dan Tian Standing position – Inhale

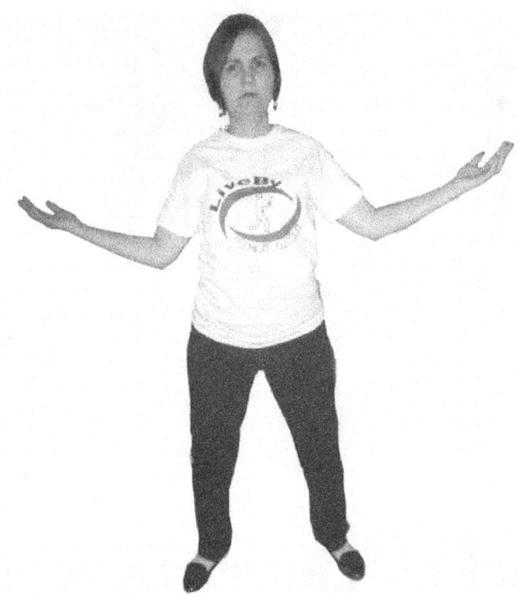

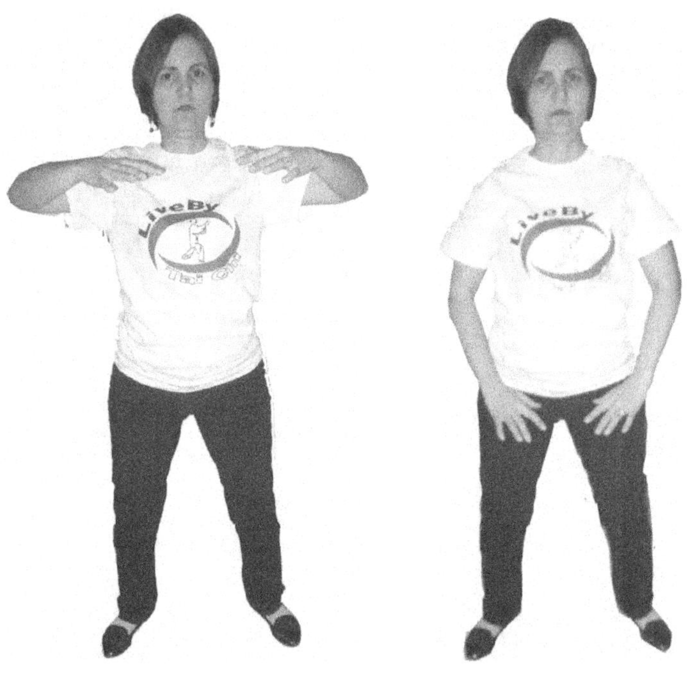

1.2 High Tide and Low Tide Arms/Hands

Objective: This rising and falling promotes gentle stimulation throughout all the tissues of your body, gently stimulating the flow of fluids, the activity of nerves and the movement of other energies within the body. This exercise is very good for mental health problems, including anxiety, depression and stress. This exercise works the anterior fibres of the deltoid, pectoralis major, biceps brachii and coracobrachialis (clavicular fibres).

How to perform:

Step 1: You start by focusing on your breathing and making it deep and slow, raising your arms on inhalation, and lowering them on exhalation.

Step 2: Breathe in as your arms come up at the level of your shoulders.

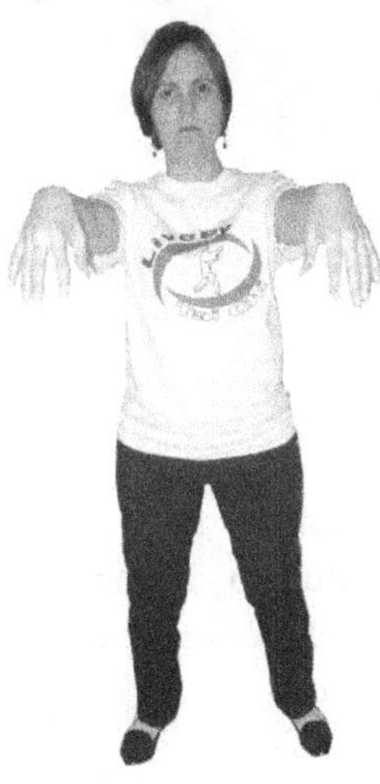

Step 3: Breathe out while your arms come down to the centre of Dan Tian or near your belly button. As your arms come down you slightly flex (bend) your knees.

- Please remember to keep the whole body relaxed.
- Check your ankles, knees, hips, back, shoulders, neck and arms as you do this so that the energy can move freely and smoothly through your body.

1.3 Pumping Hands

Objective: To relax upper body and to improve hand grip.

How to perform:

Step 1: Bend your elbows and make a fist with both hands. Make a fist and place your thumb against the knuckles of your index and middle fingers. Then, squeeze your fist a little like you are holding all the tension in your body.

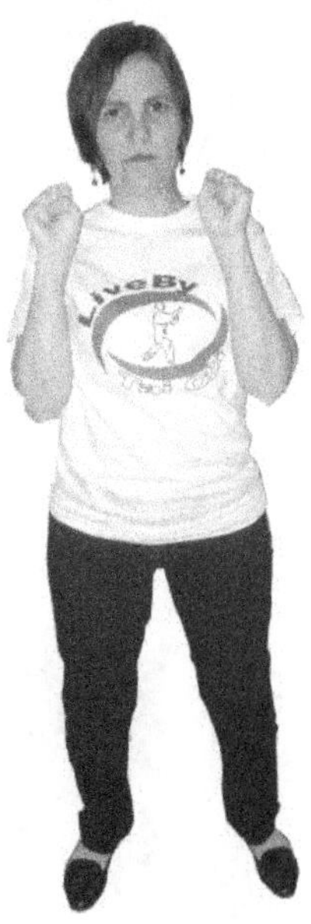

Step 2: Extend (straighten) your elbow and hand down. Palms pointed to the floor. Breathe out and let all tension release.

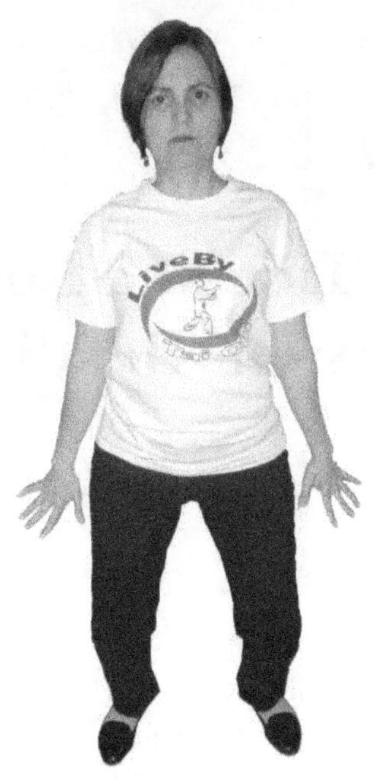

2. Neck

2.1 High Tide and Low Tide with Neck Flexion (Bending Forward)

Objective: To improve neck posture. Strengthening these muscles can help improve posture and get the head closer to neutral position. To reduce neck pain related to poor posture. This exercise strengthens the muscles that pull the head back into alignment over the shoulders (upper thoracic extensors and the deep cervical flexors.) This exercise works anterior fibres of the deltoid, pectoralis major, biceps brachii and coracobrachialis (clavicular fibres).

How to perform:

Step 1: Concentrate on the breathing principles. You start by simply focusing on your breathing and making it deep and slow, raising your arms on inhalation, and lowering them on exhalation.

Step 2: Breathe in as your arms come up at the level of your shoulders.

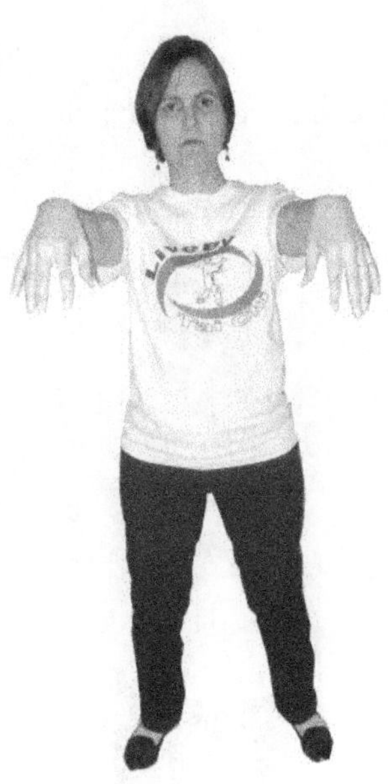

Step 3: Breathe out while your arms come down to the centre of Dan Tian or near your belly button. As your arms come down slightly flex (bend) your knees.

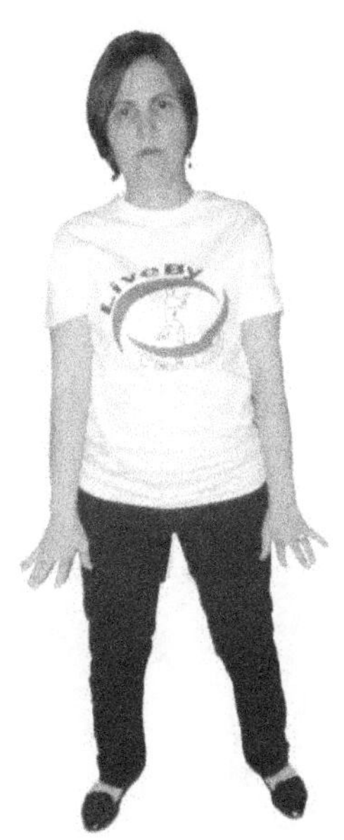

Step 4: Breathe out and bring your arms down slowly and move your head down.

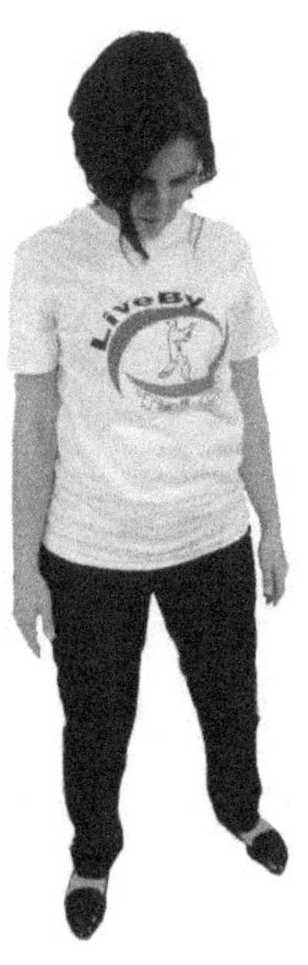

Step 5: Then, return to the starting position and look in front of you with your chin tucked.

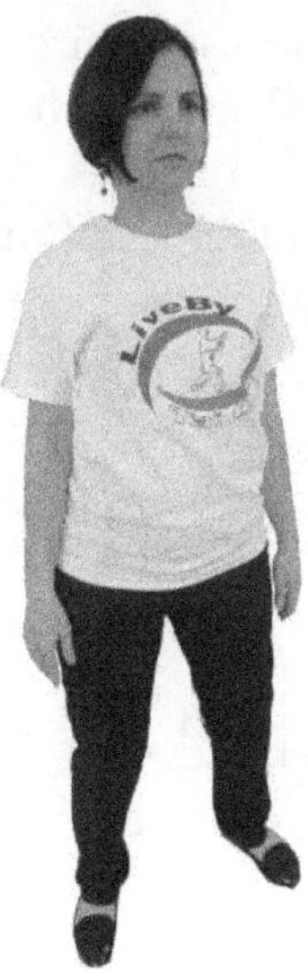

- Please remember to keep the whole body relaxed.
- Check your ankles, knees, hips, back, shoulders, neck and arms as you do this so that the energy can move freely and smoothly through your body.

2.2 Chin Tuck and Nerve Mobilization

Objective: To improve neck posture. Strengthening these muscles can help improve posture and get the head closer to neutral position. This exercise strengthens the muscles that pull the head back into alignment over the shoulders (upper thoracic extensors and the deep cervical flexors.) The push movement promotes mobilization of the nerves.

How to perform:

Step 1: Stand naturally and relaxed with your feet shoulder width apart, nice and tall, and slightly bend your knees to ease pressure on your hips.

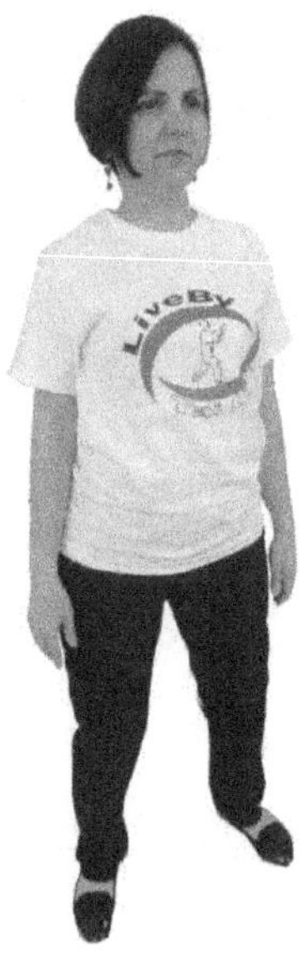

Step 2: Lift your arms until they are about shoulder height (breathing in). Your arms need to float in front of your body.

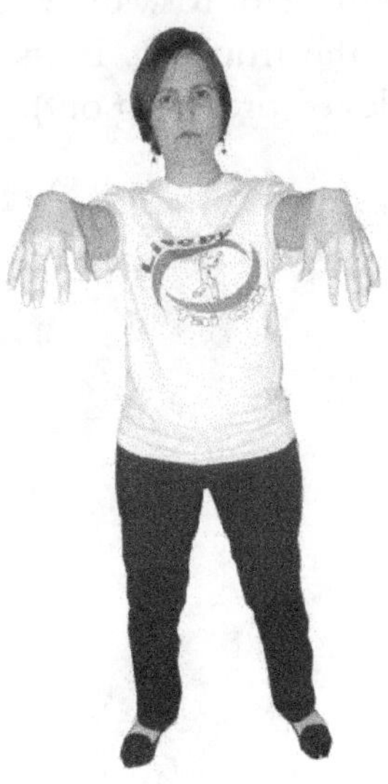

Step 3: Turn your palms to face yourself, bend your elbow and bring your hands towards your shoulders. When you bring your arms towards yourself, perform a chin tuck by moving your chin back and gently down to align your ears with your shoulders. You should feel a stretch in the back of your neck (turtle posture- neck retraction).

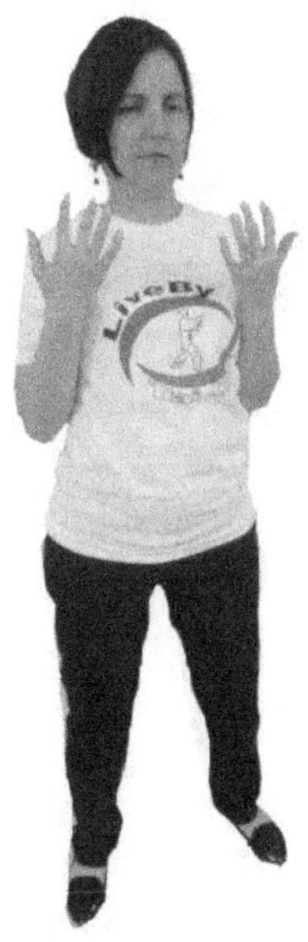

Step 4: Turn your palm and let the back of your hands to face you, then extend your elbow (similar to a stop sign). Bring one leg to the front and bend your knee while you lean forward and transfer around eighty percent of your weight to the front leg. Press out with your hands and relax and lower your shoulders (breathing out).

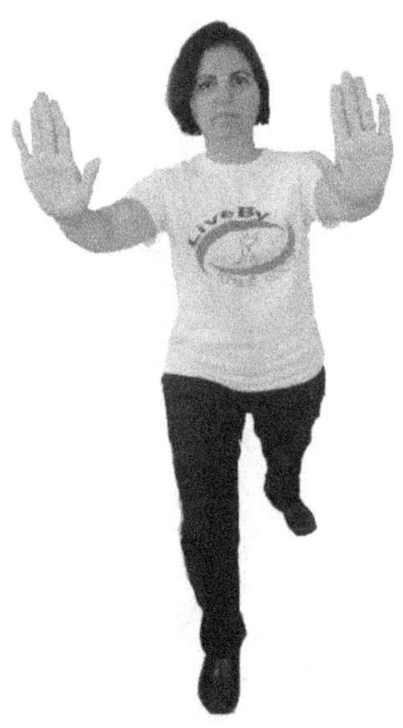

Step 5: Then, back to Step 3 and repeat the same, alternating your legs each time that you lean forward.

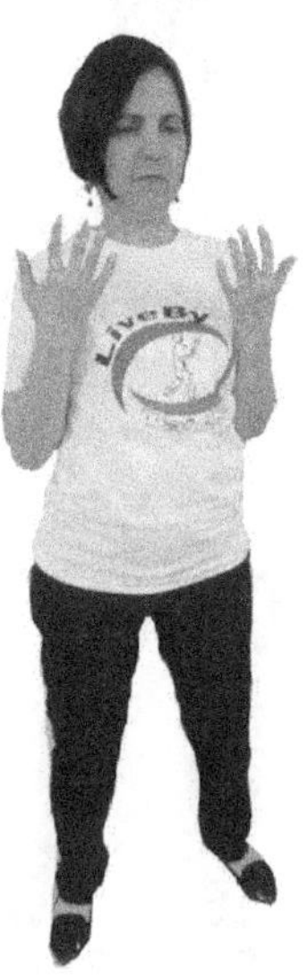

2.3 Neck Rotation- Cloudy Hands

Objective: To improve neck posture. This exercise stretches the muscles that rotate your cervical spine, turning the head to the left or to the right. It promotes rotary movement around the longitudinal axis of the bone. Muscles involved in this exercise: Sternocleidomastoid, obliquus capitis inferior, obliquus capitis superior, rectus capitis lateralis, longissimus capitis, splenius capitis, semispinalis capitis and trapezius (upper fibers). Relieves tension on the upper and lower body, improves co-ordination of upper and lower body; excellent to improve balance and transfer body weight side to side; improves flexibility of neck and shoulder; improves breathing and relieves anxiety. This exercise also improves hip flexibility and works well for lateral weight transfer.

How to perform:

Step 1: Stand naturally and relaxed with your feet shoulder width apart. Stand nice and tall, and slightly bend your knees to ease pressure on your hips. You start by standing or sitting with a straight back posture. Position your hands as though you are holding an "imaginary ball".

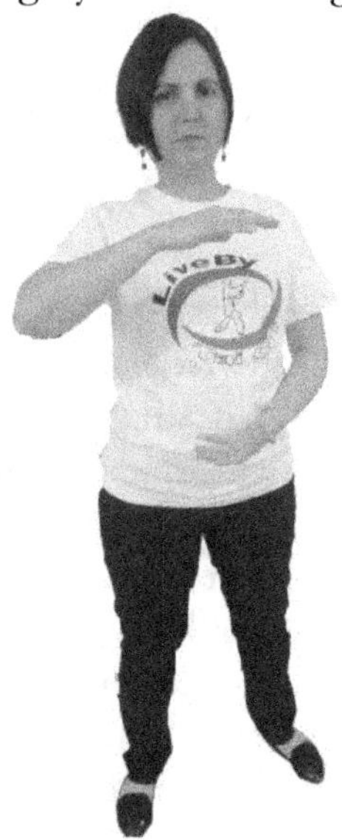

Step 2: Bend your knees and relax your arms.

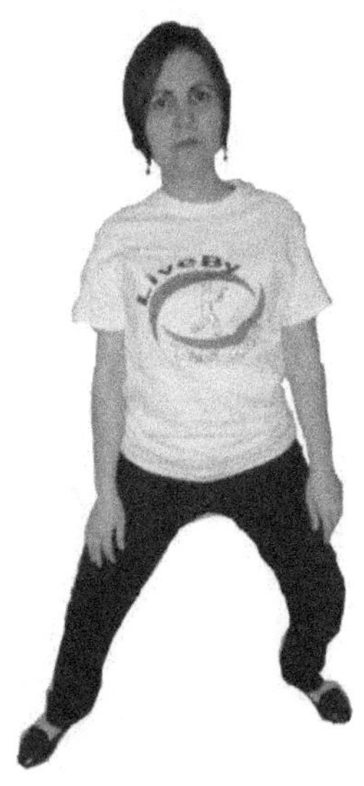

Step 3: Bring one hand to the opposite side of your face. Hand up with your palm towards yourself, as though you are looking at yourself in the mirror.

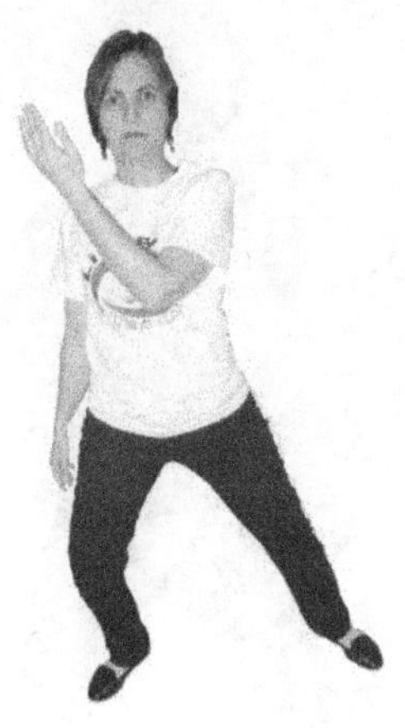

Step 4: Slide hand down across your body and transfer your weight to the side on which your hand is up.

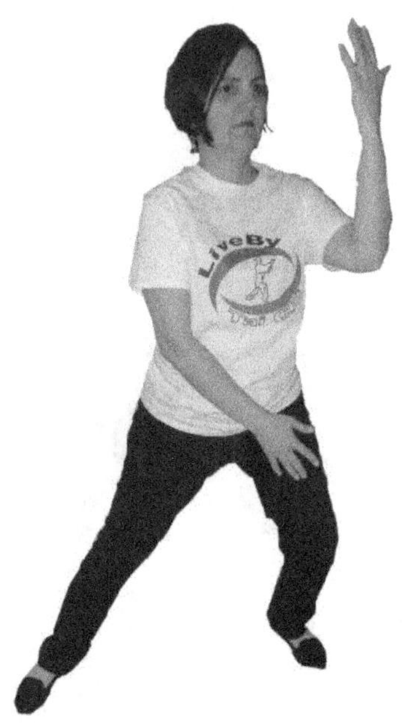

Step 5: Switch your hands and transfer your weight to the other side. The hand that was up goes down and the hand that was down goes up. Repeat this posture using opposite hand in Step 3.

2.4 Neck Lateral Flexion and Nerve Mobilization (Stop Sign)

Objective: To stretch and mobilize cervical spine and nerves. This exercise is excellent for carpal tunnel syndrome and neck pain.

How to perform:

Step 1: Stand naturally and relaxed with your feet shoulder width apart. Stand nice and tall, and slightly bend your knees to ease pressure on your hips. Bring your hand to the level of your shoulders at 90 degrees. Relax your hands in a flexed position. Your fingers are pointed down to the floor.

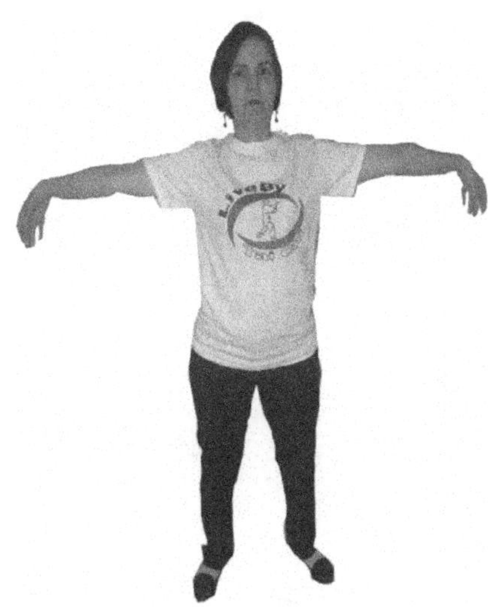

Step 2: Extend your wrist, like you are doing a "stop" sign on both sides of your arms. Try to keep your elbow straight, but if you feel numbness or tingling you can bend your elbow slightly.

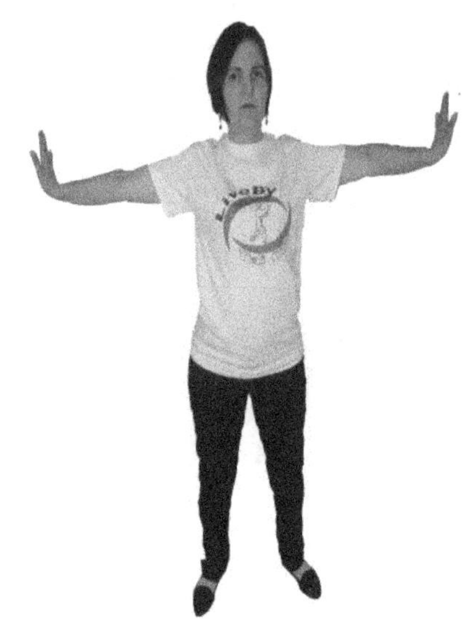

Step 3: Bend your head to one side.

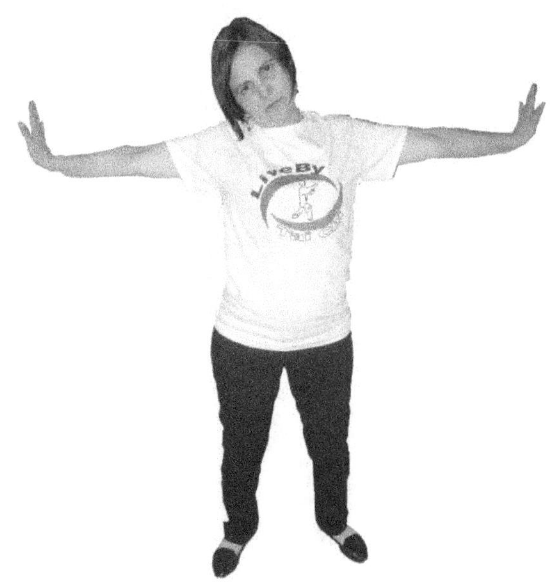

Step 4: Then, gently move your head up and down on the side. Do not extend your head too much (neck backward). Movements should be very slow and gentle. Repeat this posture bending to opposite side in Step 3.

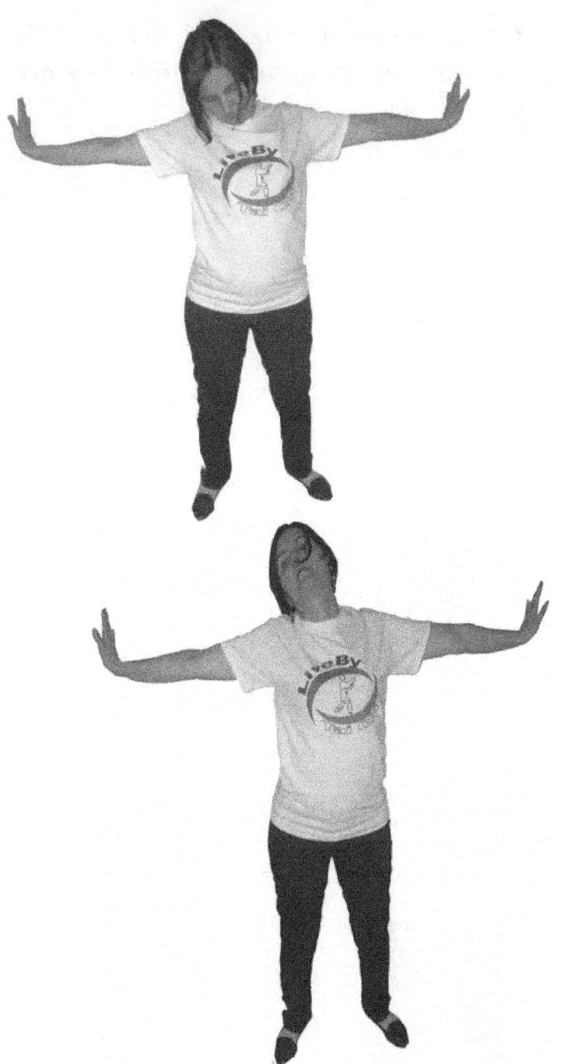

2.5 Neck Lateral Flexion and Nerve Mobilization (Holding needles)

Objective: To stretch and mobilize cervical spine and nerves. This exercise is excellent for nerve entrapment syndrome and to reduce neck pain.

How to perform:

Step 1: Stand naturally and relaxed with your feet shoulder width apart. Stand nice and tall, and slightly bend your knees to ease pressure on your hips. Bring your hands to the level of your shoulders at 90 degrees. Relax your hands in a flexed position. Your fingers are pointed down to the floor.

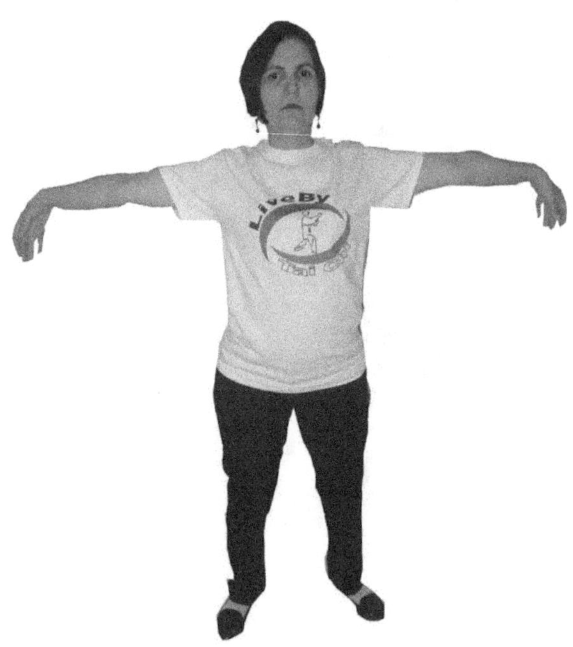

Step 2: Touch the tip of your thumb to the tip of your index finger with the others fingers relaxed. Perform a "Mudra of knowledge" (Gyan Mudra) position of the yoga with your thumb and index. This position helps to increase energy to memory power, prevents insomnia and shapes the brain.

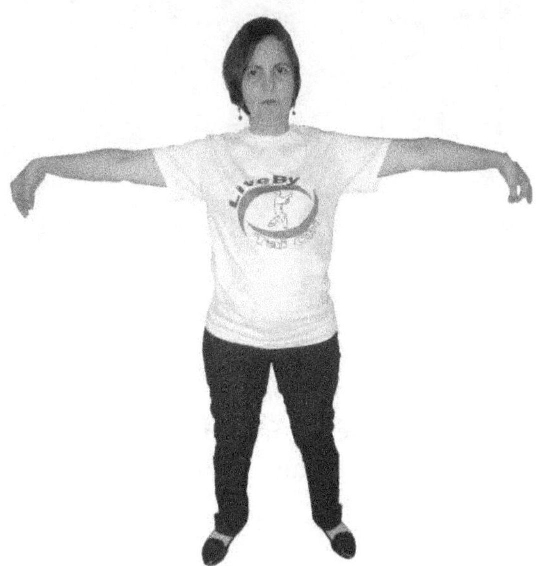

Step 3: Turn your palms up with your thumb and index finger in the same position.

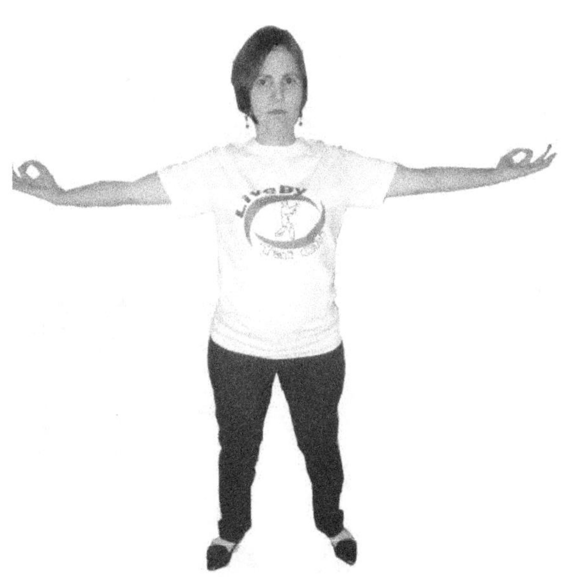

Step 4: Keep your hands in this position and bend your head to one side.

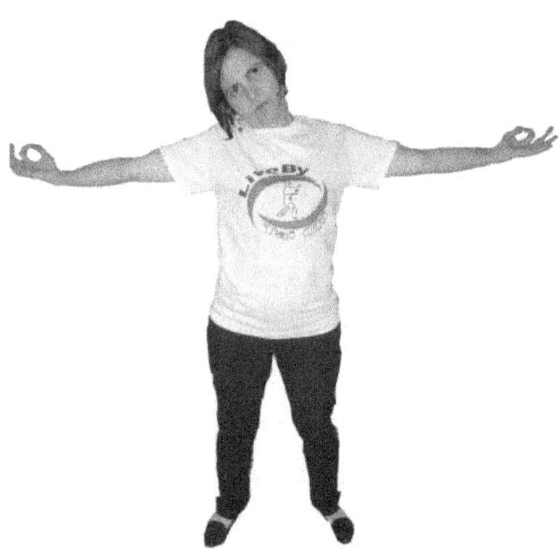

Step 5: Then, gently move your head up and down on the side. Do not extend your head too much (neck backward). Movements should be very slow and gentle. Repeat this posture bending head to opposite side in Step 4

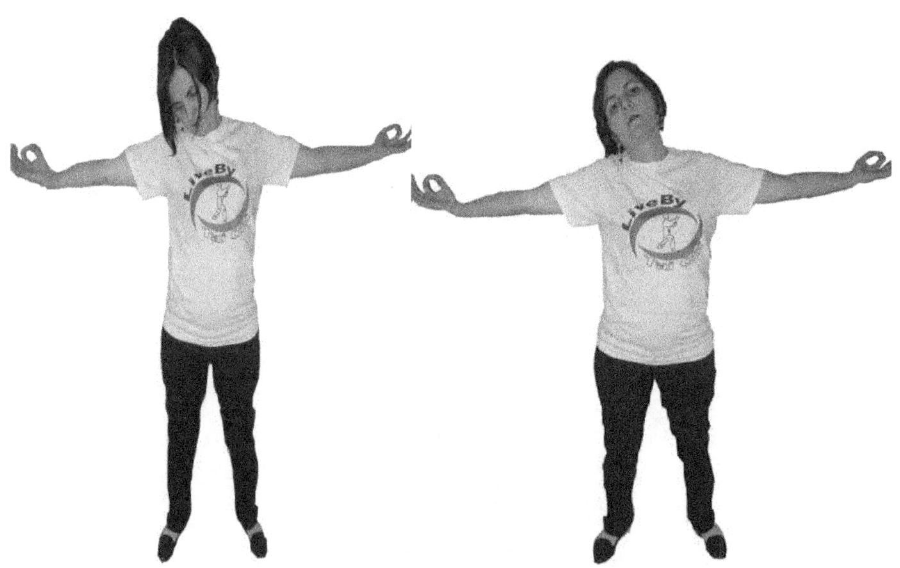

3.Shoulder

3.1 Roll Shoulder Forward and Backward

Objective: To mobilize the shoulders. This exercise is excellent for shoulder pain. It helps to relax stress, reduce stiffness of muscles and tendons, improve circulation of the shoulder and improve range of motion. You will primarily work the shoulder muscles and secondarily work the chest and upper back muscles.

How to perform:

Step 1: Stand naturally and relaxed with your feet shoulder width apart, nice and tall, and slightly bend your knees to ease pressure on your hips with your arms by your sides.

Step 2: Slowly rotate your shoulder forward, making circles

Step 3: Then, slowly rotate your shoulder backwards, making circles.
   Keep your body and mind relaxed and breathe deeply and keep the movement smooth and continuous.

3.2 Shoulder Centralization

Objective: To mobilize the shoulders and arms. This exercise is excellent for shoulder pain. It helps to relax stress, reduce stiffness of muscles and tendons, improve circulation of the shoulder and improve range of motion. In addition to these benefits, this exercise helps with your concentration and focus.

How to perform:

Step 1: Stand naturally and relaxed with your feet shoulder width apart. Stand nice and tall, and slightly bend your knees to ease pressure on your hips. Relax your arms by your side with elbow slightly flexed (bent) to keep your arms making a "semicircle". Place your hands one on the top of the other with fingers relaxed and palms up without touching each other.

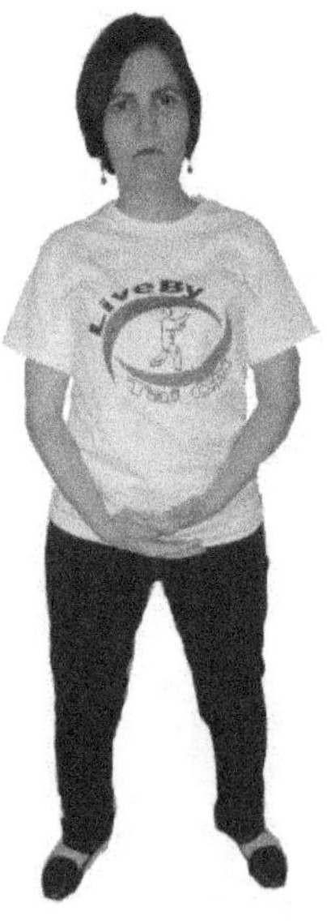

Step 2: "Open" one arm to the same side of body with your elbow slightly bent and under the level of your shoulder (around 75-80 degrees of shoulder abduction), palm facing up.

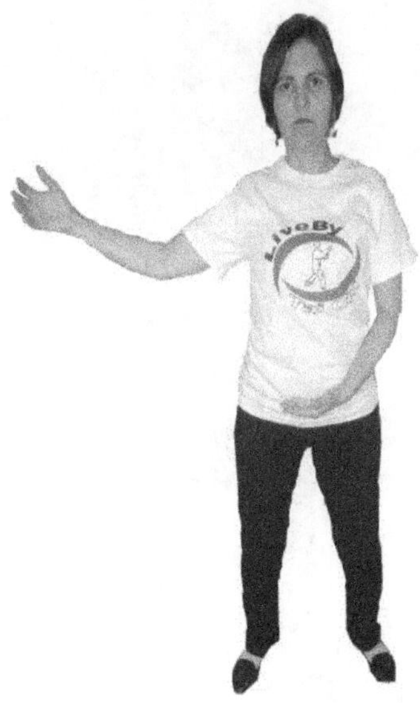

Step 3: Bring your hand to the front of your head at your body's midline with your wrist in extension.

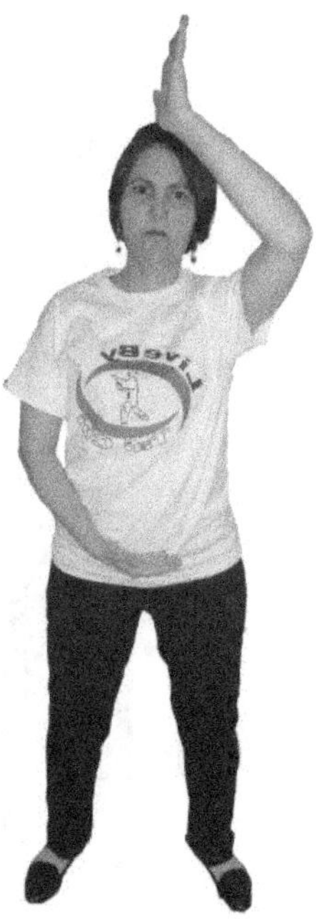

Step 4: Slowly bring your hand down following your body's midline with the wrist in extension. Repeat this posture using opposite arm in Step 2.

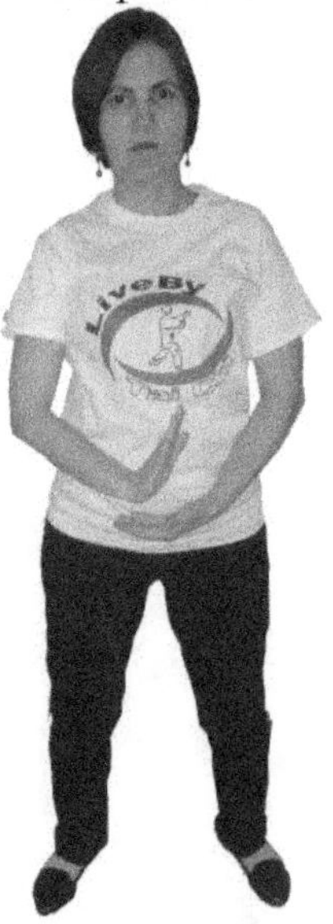

3.3 Shoulder - Hungry Bear Coming Out of Hibernation

Objective: To improve posture. To relax shoulders and neck and to work pectoral (chest) muscles. You are also working your anterior deltoids (shoulders), triceps brachii, and latissimus dorsi (back).

How to perform:

Step 1: Hands come up, elbows bend and arms placed towards your chest with hands towards your face. Squeeze your arms together.

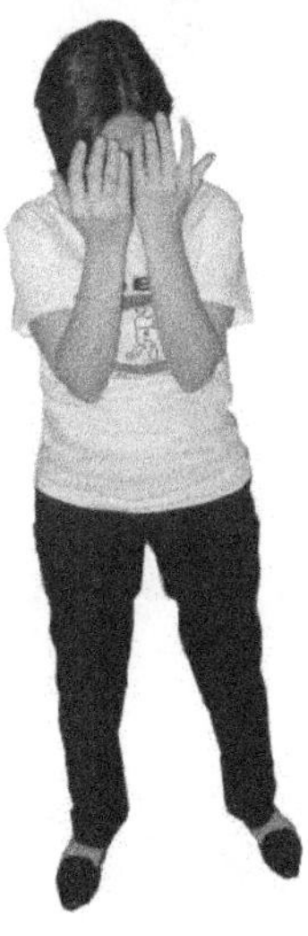

Step 2: Open chest and stretch arms behind you. You contract your upper back muscles and stretch your chest muscles.

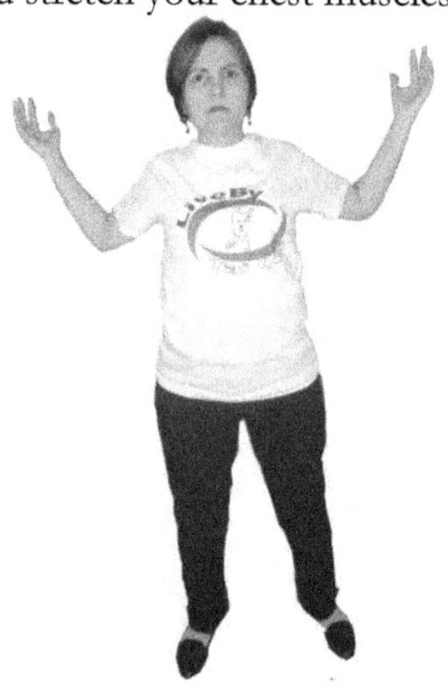

4.1 Push In and Out

Objective: To help relieve pain from carpal tunnel syndrome. This exercise promotes nerve mobilization or nerve "flossing". Nerve flossing is basically moving the nerve to try and free it from tight muscles or scar tissue that has caused it to stick to other tissues. This exercise can be used to treat tingling, pain, and burning sensations that you may have in your hand

How to perform:

Step 1:

Bend your elbows and bring your arms towards your shoulder with your palms facing your shoulders (breathing in). Turn your palm and let the back of your hands face you, then extend your elbow (similar to a stop sign). Press out with your hands and relax and lower your shoulders (breathing out).

Step 2: Push your arms with straight elbows forward at the level of your shoulders with palms facing away from yourself. You extend your wrists (similar to a stop sign). Press out with your hands and relax and lower your shoulders (breathing out).

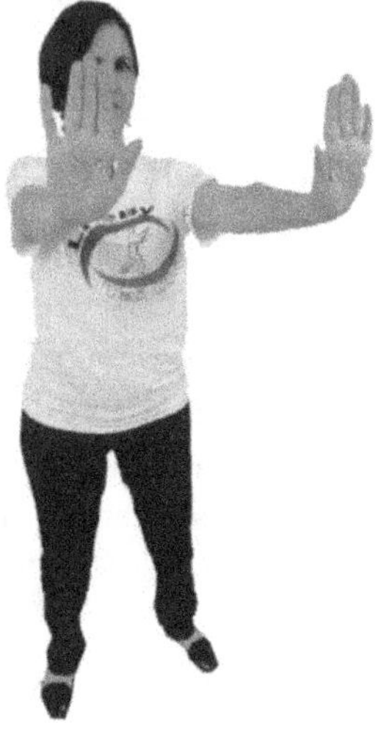

4.2 Strong Tiger

Objective: To relieve tension and anxiety. To improve hand and finger movements. To relieve pain from arthritis. To stretch your pectoralis muscles.

How to perform:

Step 1: Bend your elbows and cross your arms in front of your chest with a Tiger Claw. This is an open hand strike, fingers splayed and bent in a claw position.

Step 2: Turn your palms away from your body.

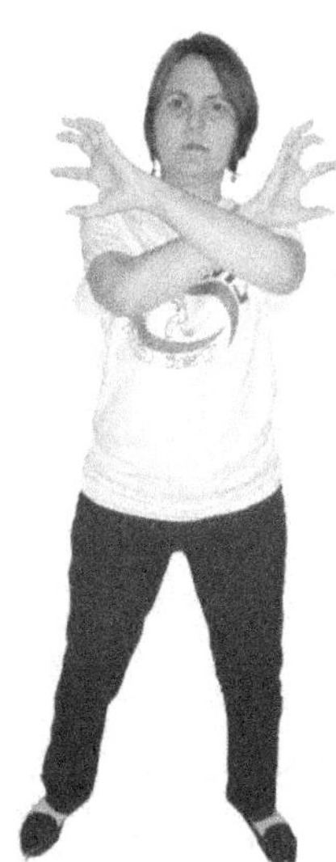

Step 3: Open your chest while you move your arms and hands to your side, until you finish in a lateral open arms position.

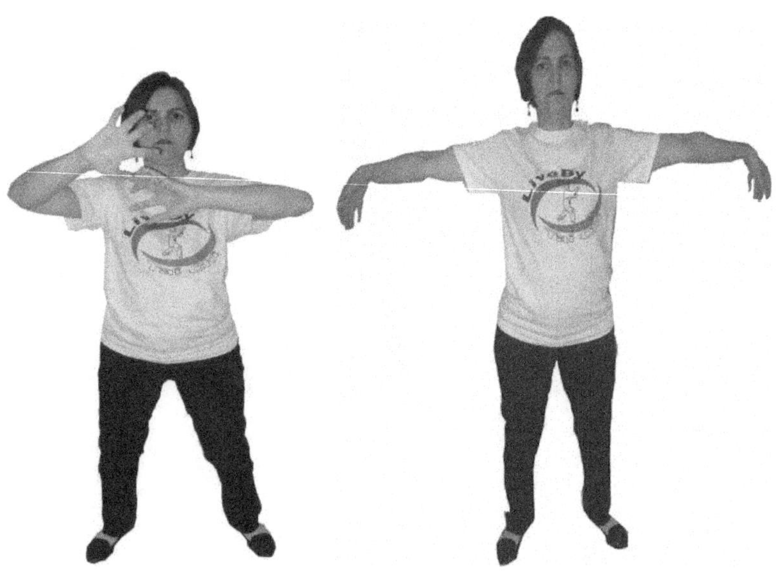

4.3 Big Circles- One Arm

Objective: To relieve tension in the upper and lower body. To improve co-ordination in upper and lower body. To improve balance and transfer of body weight. To improve flexibility of neck and shoulders. To relieve anxiety.

How to perform:

Step 1: Stand naturally and relaxed with your feet shoulder width apart. Put one arm out to your side.

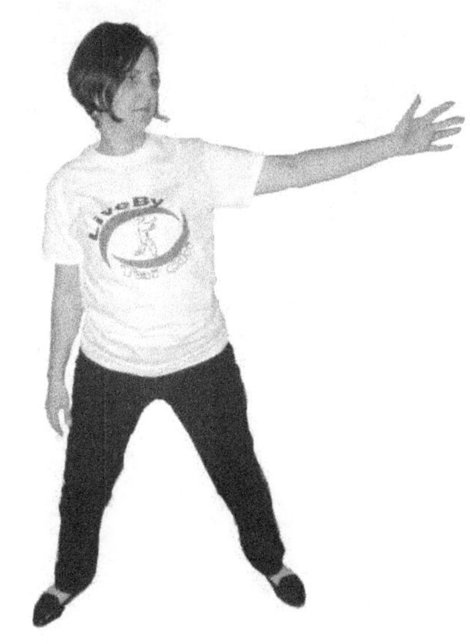

Step 2: Slide your arm down and make a big circle with your arm in front of you. At the same time you bend your knee and turn to the opposite side of your body. Let your head and face follow the direction of the movement of your arm. Then, repeat this posture with other arm in Step 1.

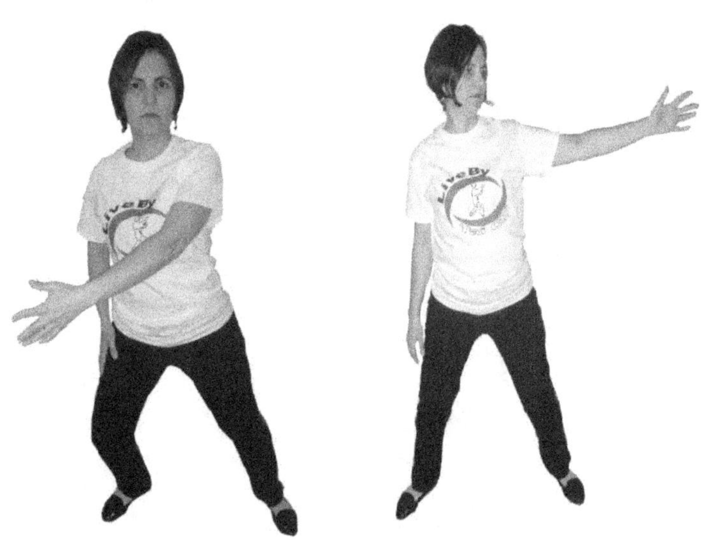

4.4 Bird Flying in the Spring

Objective: To relieve tension on the upper arm and median nerve. To improve flexibility of arms and hands.

How to perform:

Step 1: Bend one elbow and bring close to your body. Have one hand in a position like holding a tray. You are pretending that you have birds in that hand.

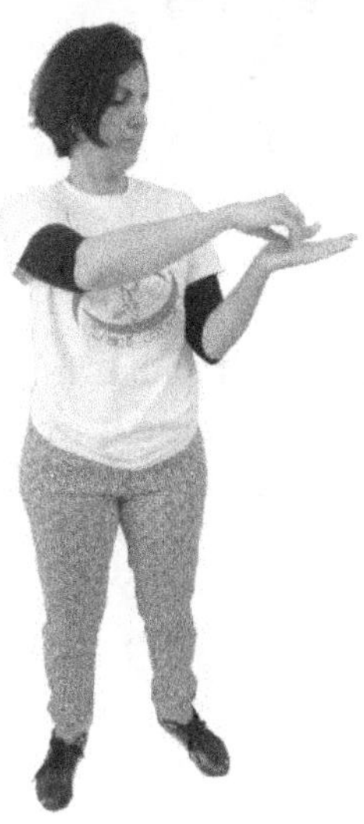

Step 2: Pretend that you are picking up a bird with your other hand and are moving the bird to your other side.

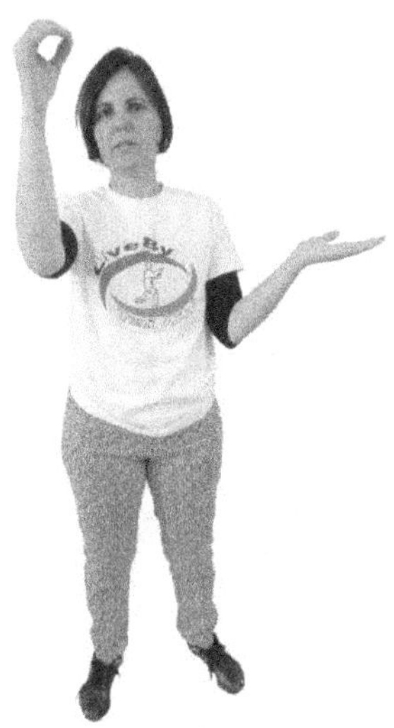

Step 3: Then, open your hand as if to let the bird fly (like you are holding a tray on your hand). At the same time, turn your head to this same side. Repeat this posture beginning in Step 1 and switch actions of hands and move to other side of body.

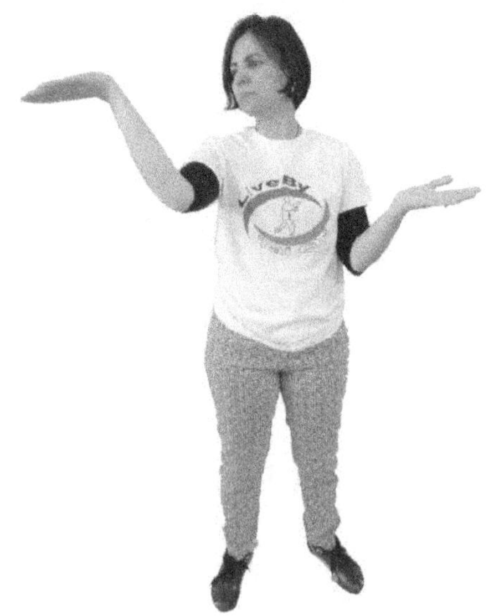

5.1 Hug Horse Stance

Objective: To relieve tension and anxiety. To improve posture and accumulate qi and energy.

How to perform:

Step 1: Inhale and exhale and bring your arms up to your shoulder's level with your elbows bent and hands towards yourself like you are hugging a big ball or a horse. You can close your eyes and keep this position for five to ten seconds.

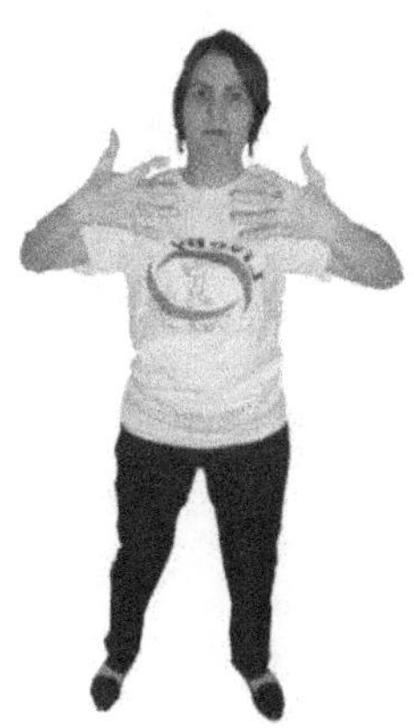

Step 2: Extend (straighten) your elbows and let hands hang down. Palms are pointed to the floor.

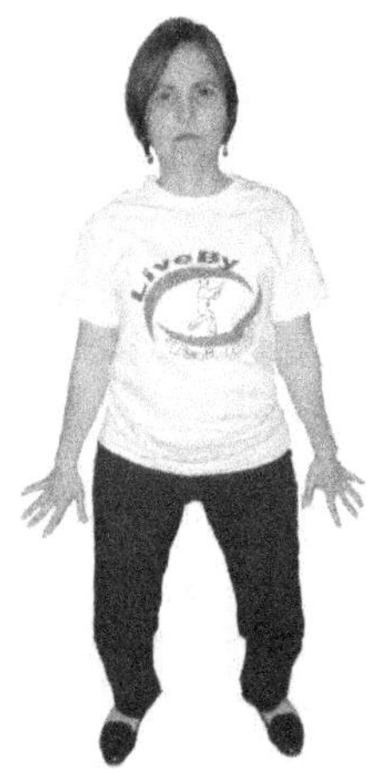

5.2 Upper Back: Front and Back Semi-Circle

Objective: To improve the strength of the middle and upper back muscles.

How to perform:

Step 1: Stand with your knees relaxed and position your hands like you are holding an imaginary ball from top to bottom and breathe in.

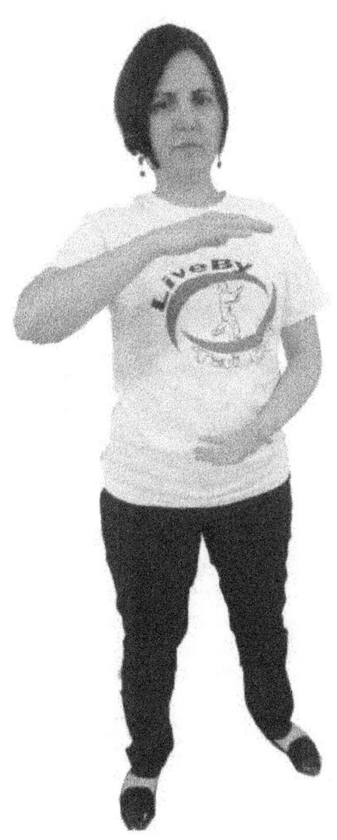

Step 2: Breathe out and move one hand up on top of your head with your palm up to the ceiling and the other hand with your palm down. Place one leg to the front (at the same side that you have your arm up). Make sure you have a good posture and feel the contraction of the muscles of your upper back. Then, switch to the other side in a circle with slow movement and switch the other leg to the front. Bend your front knee and the other arm moves up.

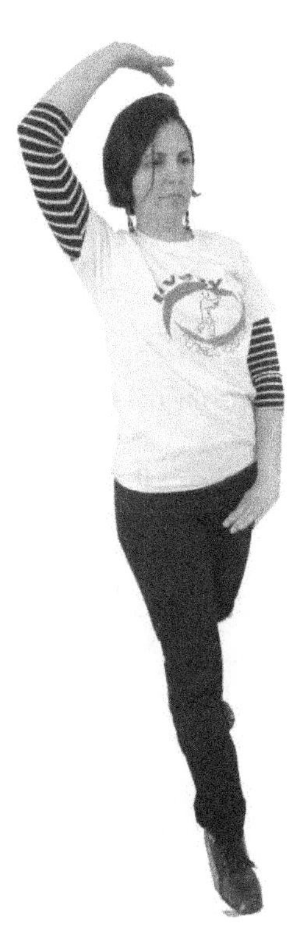
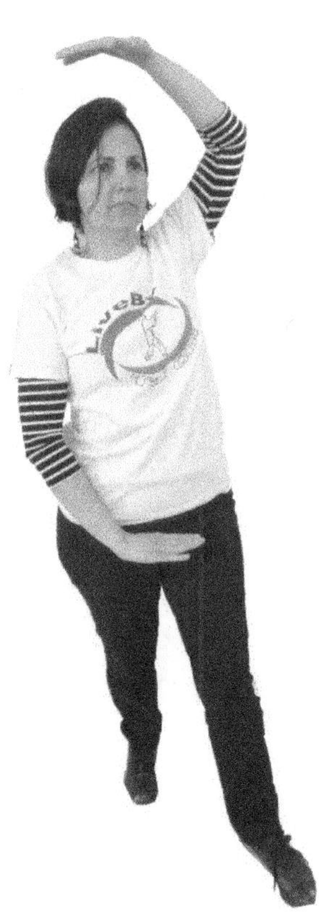

5.3 Opening and Closing Hands

Objective: To improve the strength of the middle and upper back muscles and to stretch the pectoralis muscle.

How to perform:
Step 1: Stand with your knees relaxed and position your hands in front of your chest. Breathe out as you push hands in towards each other like you are holding an imaginary ball.

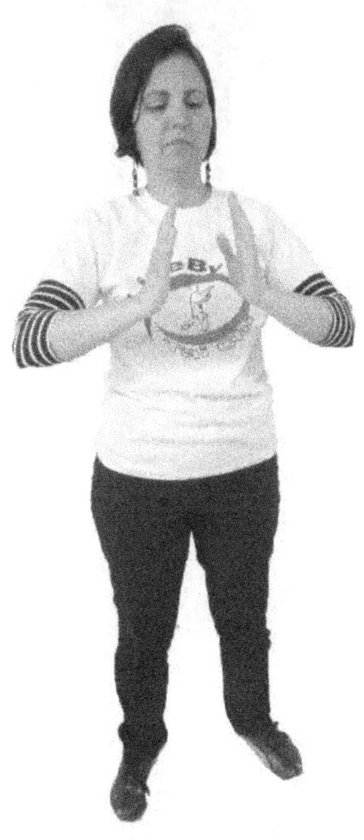

Step 2: Breathe in as you open your hands to your side with elbows bent.

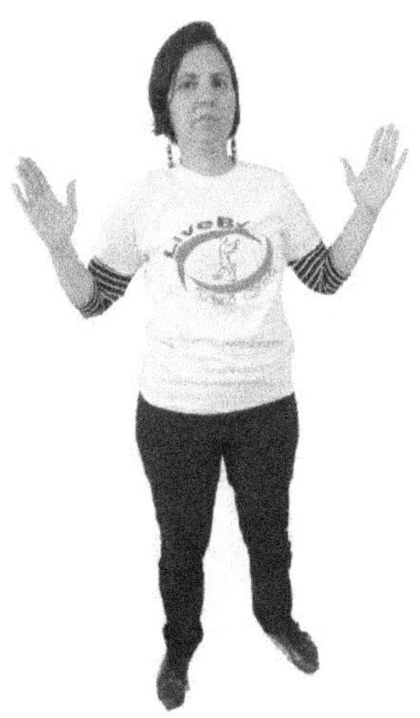

5.4 Spine Twist in Low Stance

Objective: To improve back flexibility and strength the knees.

How to perform:

Step 1: Stand with knees bent in a lower stance and position your hand like you are holding an imaginary ball top to bottom and breathe in.

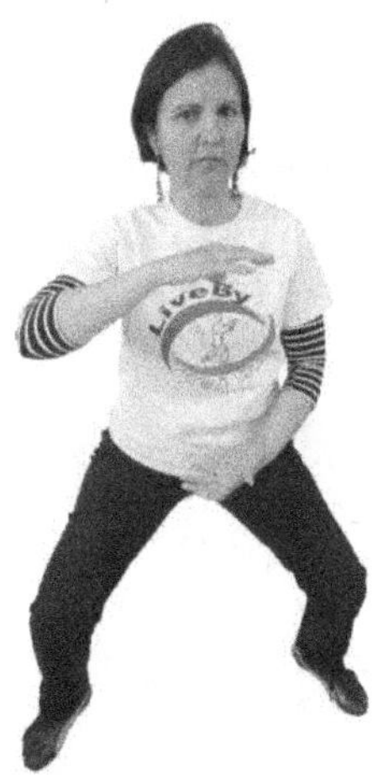

Step 2: Turn your body to one side without moving your feet, then alternate the position of your hands. The hand that is up goes down and the other hand that is down goes up, like you are turning a ball in your hands.

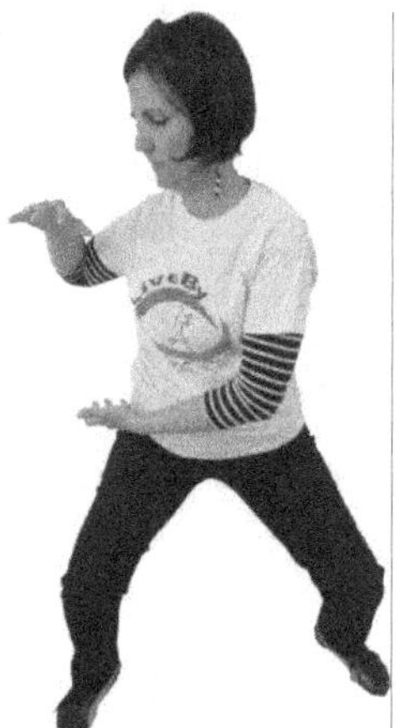

Step 3: Then, turn to the other side of your body and turn the "ball" again.

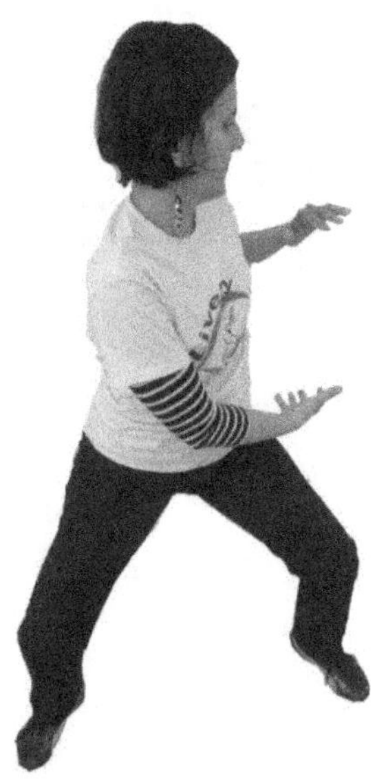

6. Hip

6.1 Hip Circle

Objective: To activate muscles around the hips and buttocks (glutes) and to stretch muscles of the pelvis.

How to perform:

Step 1: Stand nice and tall and bend your knees. Let your right knee slowly lower to the right, keeping your left leg and your pelvis in place. Then move to the opposite side making a circle (left). Then make the circle to the other side.

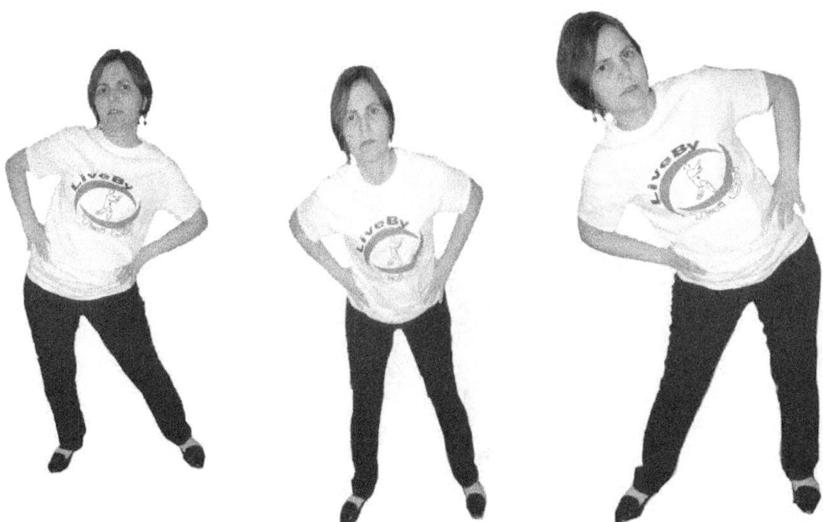

6.2 Hip Flexion (bending) and Abduction & Adduction (in/out to side)

Objective: To activate hip mobility (abduction, adduction and flexion), agility and balance.

How to perform:

Step 1: Stand nice and tall with your knees gently bent.

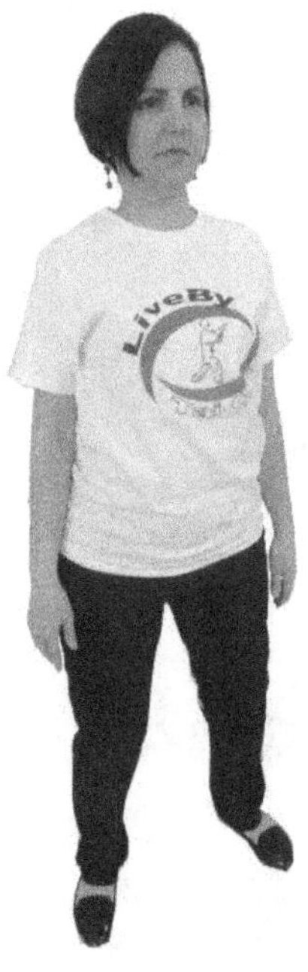

Step 2: Bring one leg up and place your hand on the same side gently on the inside of your knee.

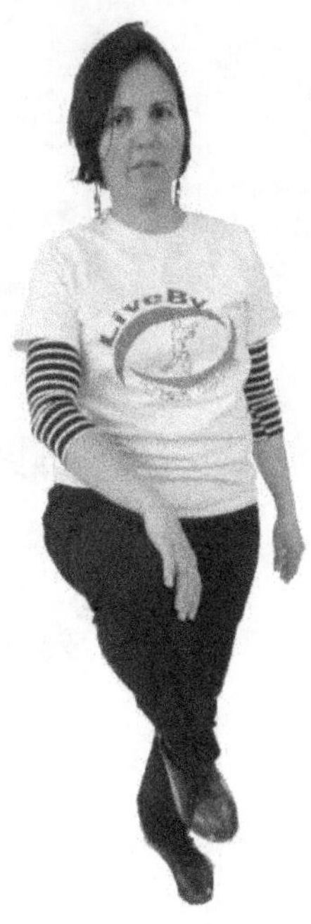

Step 3: Gently open your leg out to the side and keep your balance, standing on one leg.

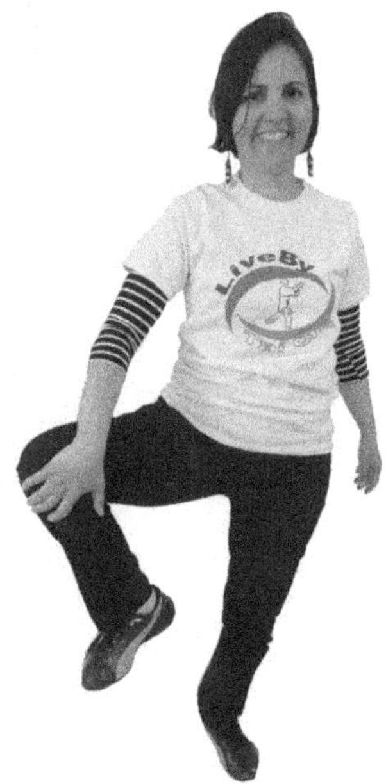

Step 4: Bring your leg back to the front, and with control, let your leg down.

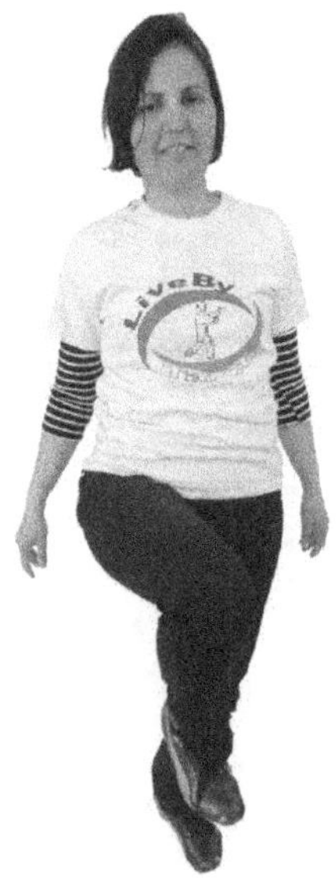

6.2 Crane Stands on One Leg

Objective: To activate hip mobility, agility, balance and gently stretch your ligaments.

How to perform:

Step 1: Stand nice and tall with feet turned out at 45 degrees. Bend your knees slightly.

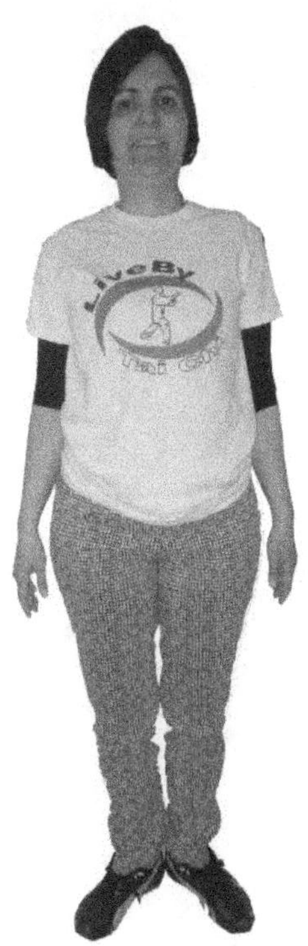

Step 2: Inhale as you raise your arms and cross them at the level of your chest with your palms towards yourself. Then, bend your knees and transfer your weight onto your right leg.

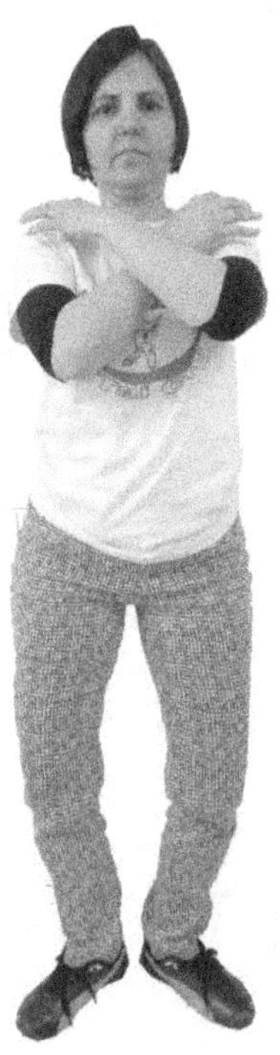

Step 3: Raise your arms with your hands moving above your head, your palms crossing each other and facing out. While you are raising your arms, lift the left knee up until it is about hip level and place your foot beside of your right knee.

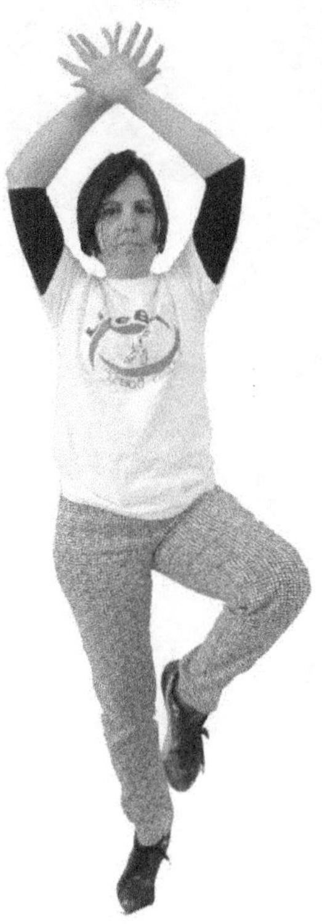

Step 4: Bring your arms to the sides of your body as you turn your palms face down with your elbows and wrists slightly bent. Keep your hands at shoulder level. Breathe out as you lower your arms back down to your sides and shift your weight onto your right leg.

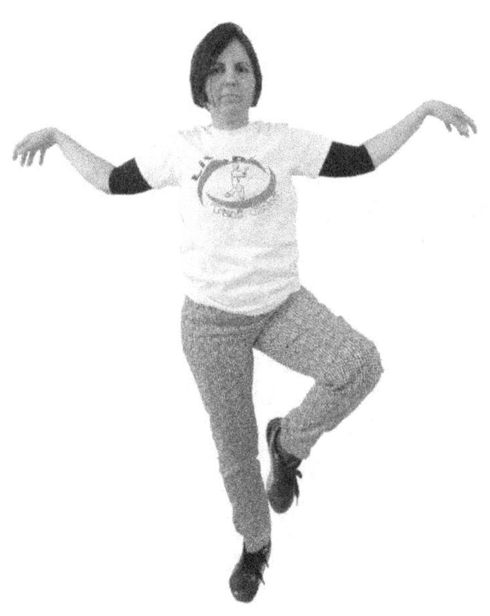

7. Knees

7.1 Prayer Wheel

Objective: To relieve tension in the upper and lower body. To improve co-ordination of upper and lower body. To improve balance and transfer of body weight. To improve flexibility of neck and shoulders. To improve breathing and to relieve anxiety.

How to perform:

Step 1: Turn your body to one side. Bring your foot on the same side that you are turning in a forward position. The back foot is at about a 45 degree angle. Then, turn your hips to face the direction of your front foot (Lunge position).

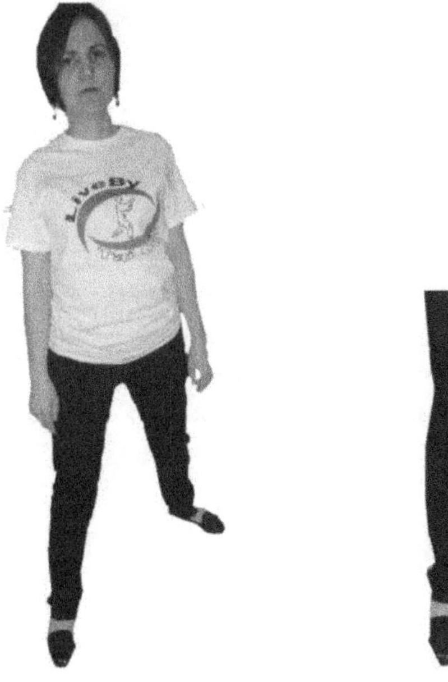

Step 2: Bend your elbows. Then place your hands out in front of you with palms facing each other. Inhale as your hands comes down to your center. Extend (straighten) your left knee and bend the right knee; making a big circle with your hands in front of you. As the hands move forward the weight is transferred around 75 to 80% more onto the front leg.

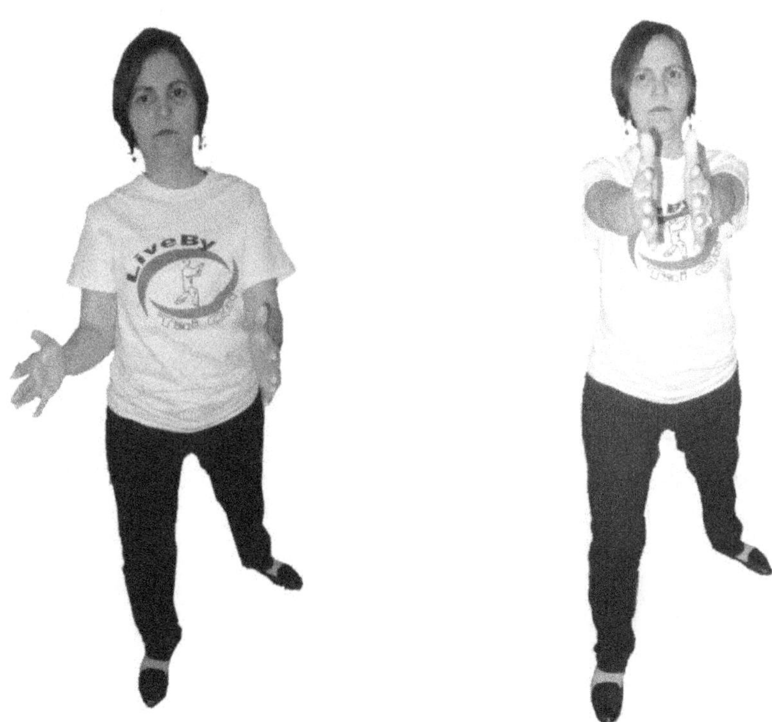

Step 3: Your hands should move in a clockwise manner in a vertical plane to trace the outline of a circle or prayer wheel, and then transfer around 75-80% of your weight to the back leg. Exhale when your arms go away from your center. Remember to keep your back heel on the floor. Repeat this posture and begin by turning body to opposite side in Step 1.

7.1 Heel Kick: Left and Right

Objective: To activate knee muscles, especially quadriceps (front thigh).

How to perform:

Step 1: Bend your knees and keep your hands in a position like you are holding a soccer ball.

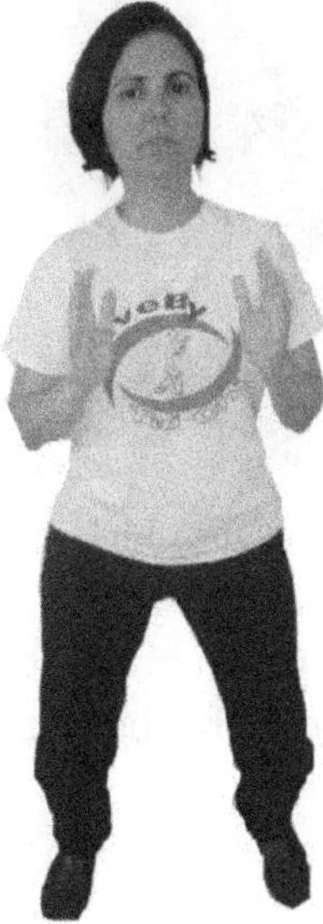

Step 2: Go up slowly by straightening your knees a little bit and stand on one leg.

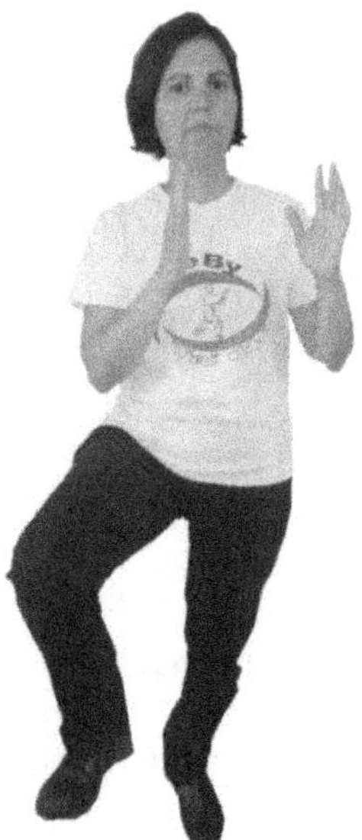

Step 3: Both palms face in at shoulder level and your elbows need to be around eighty percent extended (straightened). Turn your leg that is up slightly out to the side and extend (straighten) your knee and at the same time open your hands with palms facing out and your elbows bent.

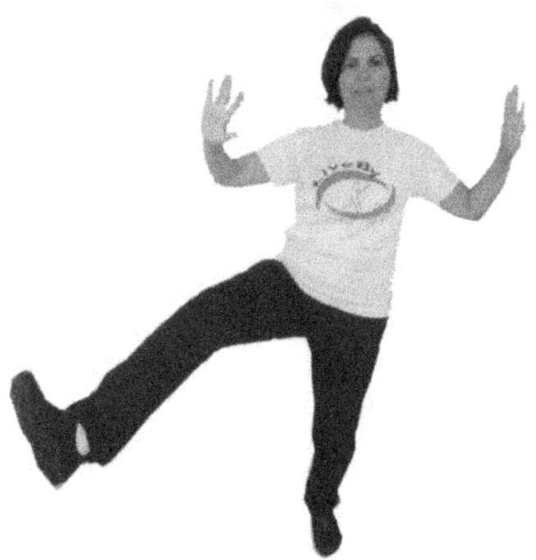

Step 4: Bend your knee and return your leg back to the front and gently put your leg down. Repeat this posture and begin by standing on opposite leg in Step 2.

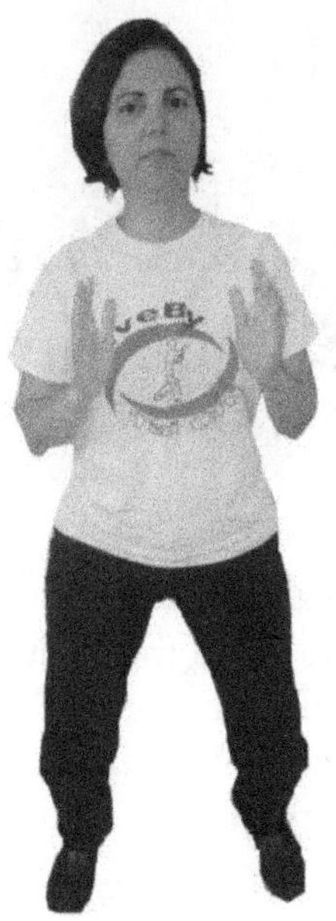

8. Ankle

8.1 Heels and Toes: Ankle Dorsiflexion & Plantar Flexion (up/down)

Objective: To improve balance and activate primary muscles that dorsiflex and plantar flex the ankle (move it up/down). (Plantaris, flexor hallucis longus, flexor digitorum longus, tibialis posterior, peroneus longus, peroneus brevis, tibialis anterior, extensor digitorum longus, extensor hallucis longus and peroneus tertius.

How to perform:

Step 1: Point your toes downward a far as you can. Hold for 3 seconds.

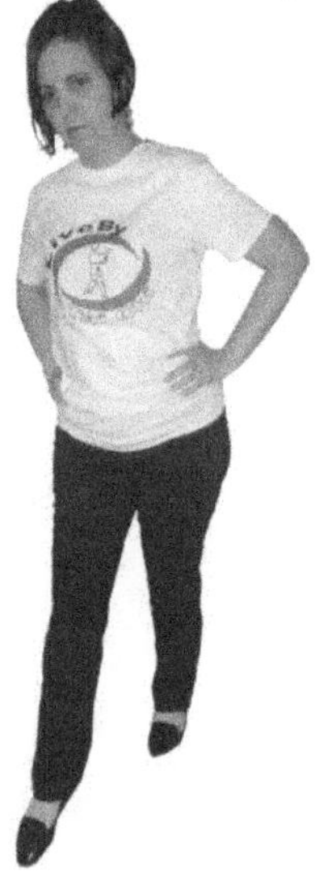

Step 2: Bend your ankle upward as far as you can. Hold for 3 seconds.

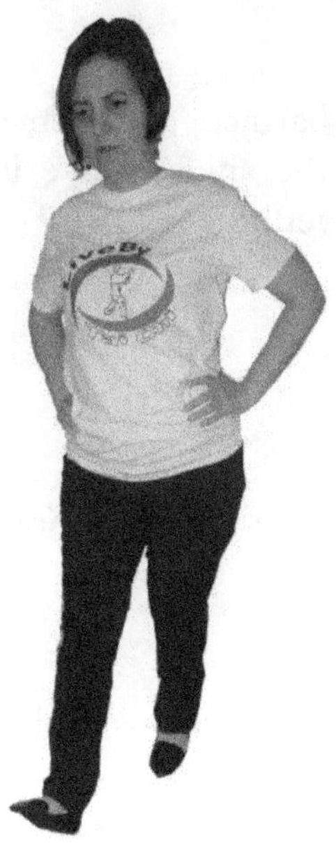

8.2 Dorsiflexion / Plantar Flexion Coordination

Objective: To improve balance and activate primary muscles that dorsiflex and plantar flex the ankle (move it up/down). Activates coordination of upper and lower body.

How to perform:

Step 1: Step your left leg to the front and point your left toes downward as far as you can.

Step 2: Bring your left arm to the opposite side with your palm facing the other side.

Step 3: Bend your right elbow and bring your hand to your center, like you are doing a stop sign. Repeat this posture beginning with right leg in Step 1 and use right arm beginning in Step 2.

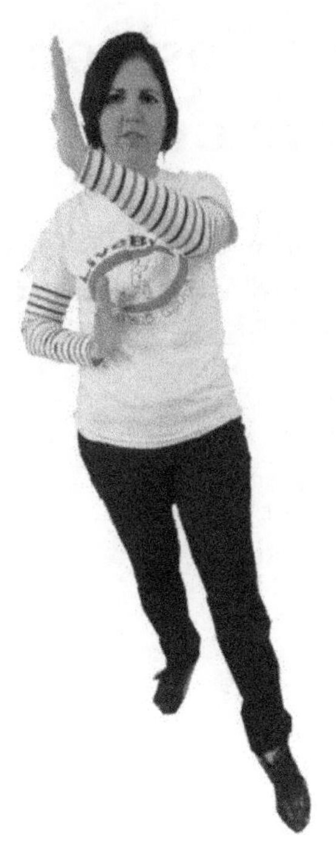 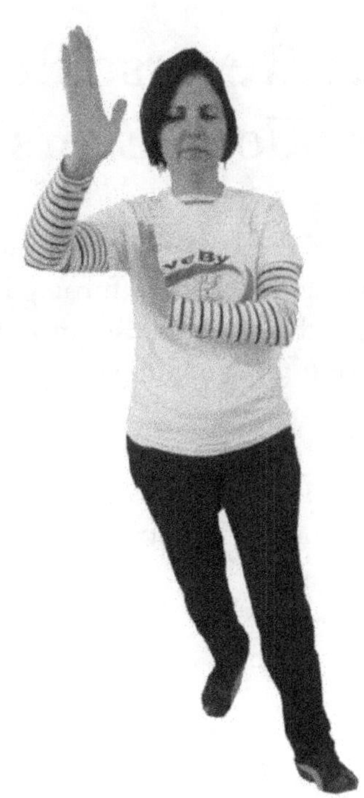

8.3 Reverse Prayer Hands Position for Foot Eversion & Inversion

Objective: To improve balance and activate the primary muscles for foot inversion/eversion (turning in/out). Activates co-ordination of upper and lower body. It is also an opportunity to perform flexibility of the wrist flexion (bending down).

How to perform:

Step 1: Step forward with one leg and place your foot in an eversion position (tilt the sole of the foot away from your body).

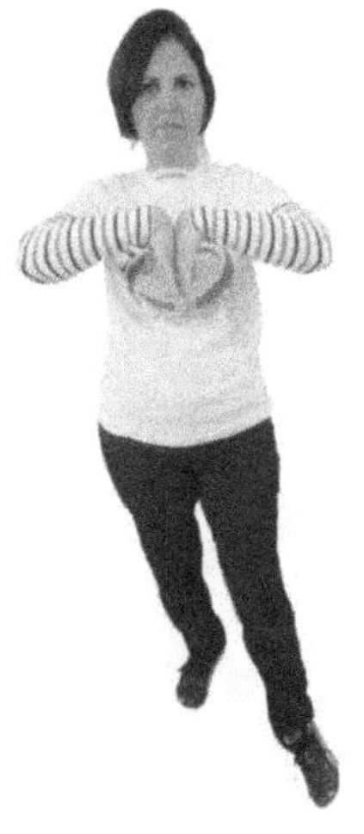

Step 2: Then, place your foot in an inversion position (tilt the sole of the foot towards your body). Repeat the two steps with other leg.

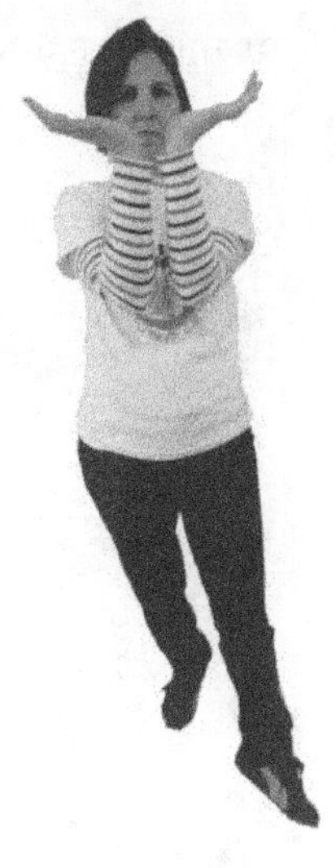

8.4 Commencement Posture Sun Style

Objective: To activate your foot muscles and work foot proprioception, balance and weight transfer.

How to perform:

Step 1: Stand nice and tall in a relaxed position.

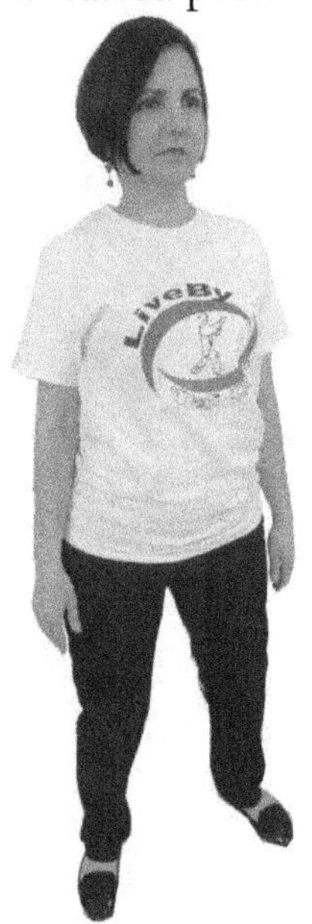

Step 2: Breathe in and raise both arms out in front of you like you are holding a ball.

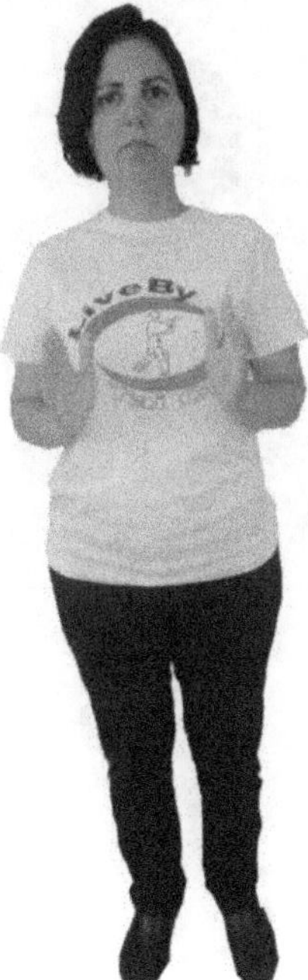

Step 3: Transfer your weight to the right leg, then, bring your right leg to the front, stepping forward with right heel.

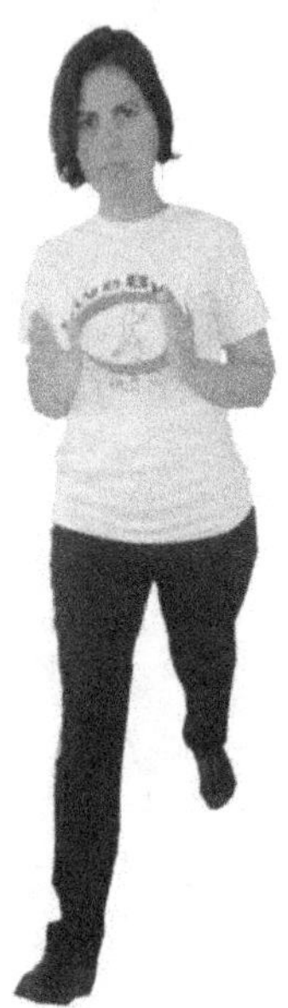

Step 4: Then flatten your foot on the floor. Bend your front knee and lean forward at the same time that you extend your elbows and bring your arms to the front and transfer around 80 percent of your weight to your front leg.

Step 5: Then bring your arms back to you like you are holding a ball.

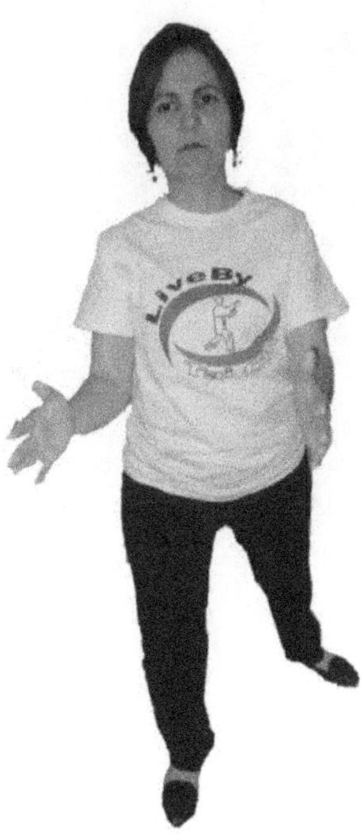

Step 6: Then, bring your arms close to you and the back leg to your front.

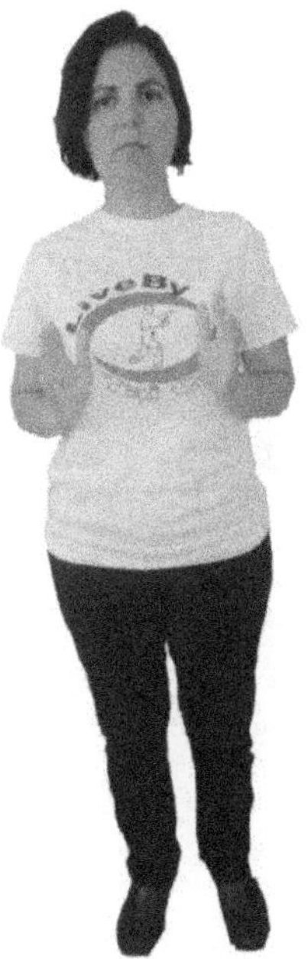

Step 7: Then, bring your arms and legs to the start position. Repeat this

posture beginning with opposite leg in Step 3.

Bibliography

A McGibbon, C., E Krebs, D., W Parker, S., M Scarborough, D., M Wayne, P., & and L Wolf, S. (2005). Tai Chi and vestibular rehabilitation improve vestibulopathic gait via different neuromuscular mechanisms: Preliminary report. BMC Neurol ; 5: 3.

Accad, M. (2016). How Western medicine lost its soul. Linacre Q. May; 83(2): 144–146.

Agrawal Y, C. J. (2009). Disorders of balance and vestibular function in US adults: data from the National Health and Nutrition Examination Survey, 2001-2004. . Arch Intern Med 169:938.

Alloway, R., Alloway, T., Magyari, P., & Floyd, S. (2016). An Exploratory Study Investigating the Effects of Barefoot Running on Working Memory. Percept Mot Skills Apr;122(2), 432-43.

Beta, M. A. (May 2018). What's the difference between Internal and External martial arts? Online forum comment], Message posted to https://martialarts.stackexchange.com/questions/104/whats-the-difference-between-internal-and-external-martial-arts?utm_medium=organic&utm_source=google_rich_qa&utm_campaign=google_rich_qa.

Burr, M. (1999). "Chen Zhen Lei : Handing Down the Family Treasure of Chen Taijiquan". Kungfu Magazine.

Carvel, P. (2017). The Tai Chi Space: How to move in Tai Chi and Qi Gong. Aeon Books.

Chen-style t'ai chi ch'uan. (2018). Available at: https://en.wikipedia.org/wiki/Chen-style_t'ai_chi_ch'uan. Ccessed on Jun 01 .

Chevalier, G. (2015). The effect of grounding the human body on mood. Psychol Rep. Apr;116(2):534-42.

Christensen, L. B. (2016). Tai Chi: The Thrue History & Principles.

(2018). Confucianism- Confucian Worldview. Available at: http://family.jrank.org/pages/317/Confucianism-Confucian-Worldview.html. Accessed on May 26.

Creel, H. G. (1970). What is Taoism? and others Studies in Chinease Cultural History. Midway Reprint.

Davidine Sim, D. G. (2002). Chen Style Taijiquan: The Source of Taiji Boxing.

Dougherty, P. (2018). Chapter 2: Somatosensory Systems. Available at: https://nba.uth.tmc.edu/neuroscience/s2/chapter02.html. Accessed on

June 29.

Dr Zai, J. (2015). Taoism and Science: Cosmology, Evolution, Morality, Health and more. Ultravisum.

Duvivier, B. M., Schaper, N. C., Koster, A., Kan, L. v., Peters, H. P., Adam, J. J., et al. (2017). Benefits of Substituting Sitting with Standing and Walking in Free-Living Conditions for Cardiometabolic Risk Markers, Cognition and Mood in Overweight Adults. Front Physiol.; 8: 353.

Field T, D. M. (2013). Tai chi/yoga reduces prenatal depression, anxiety and sleep disturbances. Complement Ther Clin Pract. Feb;19 (1), 6-10.

Frantzis, B. (2018). The Eight Principles of Tai Chi Chuan. Available at:
https://www.energyarts.com/sites/default/files/Tai_Chi_Eight_Principl es_Report.pdf. Acessed on May 29, 2018.

Gaétan Chevalier, 1. 2., Oschman, J. L., Sokal, K., & Sokal, a. P. (2012). Earthing: Health Implications of Reconnecting the Human Body to the Earth's Surface Electrons. J Environ Public Health. 291541.

Galante, L. (1981). Tai Chi: The Supreme Ultimate. Boston, MA/York Beach, ME: WeiserBooks.

Guang Yi, R. (2003). Taijiquan: Chen 38 form and applications. . North Clarendon VT: Tuttle Publishing.

Haselager, W. F., Broens, M., & Gonzalez, M. E. (2012). The importance of sensing one's movements in the world for the sense of personal identity. Rivista Internazionale di Filosofia e Psicologia 3, 1–11 10.

Jacobson BH, C. H. (1997). The effect of T'ai Chi Chuan training on balance, kinesthetic sense, and strength. Percept Mot Skills; 84: 15.27-33.

James A. Mortimer, D. D. (2012). Changes in Brain Volume and Cognition in a Randomized Trial of Exercise and Social Interaction in a Community-Based Sample of Non-Demented Chinese Elders. Journal of Alzheimer's Disease, Vol. 30 Number 4, 757-766.

Julia J. Tsuei. (1978). Eastern and Western Approaches to Medicine. West J Med, Jun 128:551-557.

K Rajeshwari, S. K. (2017). Evaluation of Resting Tongue Position in Recently Extracted and Long Term Completely Edentulous Patients: A Prospective Interventional Study. Journal of Clinical and Diagnostic Research. Apr, Vol-11(4), 61-63.

Kathryn M. Sibley, S. E. (2011). Balance Assessment Practices and Use of Standardized Balance Measures Among Ontario Physical Therapists. Phys Ther. Nov; 91(11): 1583–1591.

King, J. (2018). Fundamental Footwork . Available at: https://www.taichiaustralia.com/articles/Fundamental_Footwork.htm. Accessed on June 10.

Koo, M. (2017). The Dance of the Tai Chi.

Lan C, L. J. (1998). 12-month Tai Chi training in the elderly: its effect on health fitness. Med Sci Sports Exerc. 30, 345-351.

Lan C, L. J. (2000). Tai Chi Chuan to improve muscular strength and endurance in elderly individuals: a pilot study. Arch Phys Med Rehabil. ; 81, 604-607.

Lee, F. H. (2011). Complementary and alternative medicine in chronic pain. Pain. 152, 28–30.

Ling Jun Kong, R. L. (2016). Tai Chi for Chronic Pain Conditions: A Systematic Review and Meta-analysis of Randomized Controlled . Scientific report, 1-9.

Liu, H. &. (2010). Tai chi as a balance improvement exercise for older adults: A systematic review. Journal of Geriatric Physical Therapy, 33(3), 103.

Lomas-Vega R, O.-G. E.-O.-P.-C. (2017). Tai Chi for Risk of Falls. A Meta-analysis. . J Am Geriatr Soc. Sep;65(9), 2037-2043.

Man-ch'ing, C. (1993). Ch'uan, Cheng-Tzu's Thirteen Treatises on T'ai Chi. North Atlantic Books.

Nafisa Saftari, L. a.-S. (2018). Ageing vision and falls: a review. J Physiol Anthropol. 37: 11.

Nima Toosizadeh, H. E. (2018). Proprioceptive impairments in high fall risk older adults: the effect of mechanical calf vibration on postural balance. Biomed Eng Online. 17: 51.

Oschman, J. L., Chevalier, G., & Brown, a. R. (2015). The effects of grounding (earthing) on inflammation, the immune response, wound healing, and prevention and treatment of chronic inflammatory and autoimmune diseases. J Inflamm Res.; 8: 83–96.

Osypiuk, K., Thompson, E., & and Wayne, P. M. (2018). Can Tai Chi and Qigong Postures Shape Our Mood? Toward an Embodied Cognition Framework for Mind-Body Research. Front. Hum. Neurosci., 01 May.

Perkins, K., Hanney, W., & Rothschild, C. (2014). The risks and benefits of running barefoot or in minimalist shoes: a systematic review. Sports Health, 6 (6), 475-80.

Peterka, R. (2001). Sensorimotor integration in human postural control. J Neurophysiol. Sep; 88(3):1097-118.

Philip-Simpson, M. (June, 1995). "A Look at Wu Style Teaching Methods". T'AI CHI The International Magazine of T'ai Chi Ch'uan . Wayfarer Publications.

Pollard, Rosenberg, Tignor, E., Clifford, & Robert. (2011). Worlds Together Worlds Apart. New York, New York: Norton.

Rainbow Tin Hung Ho, c. a.-Y. (2014). The psychophysiological effects of Tai-chi and exercise in residential Schizophrenic patients: a 3-arm randomized controlled trial. BMC Complement Altern Med.; 14: 364.

Rosario, J., Bezerra-Diógenes, M., Mattei, R., & Leite, J. (2014). Differences and similarities in postural alterations caused by sadness and depression. J Bodyw Mov Ther. Oct;18(4):540-4.

Scheffer AC, S. M. (2008). Fear of falling: Measurement strategy, prevalence, risk factors and consequences among older persons. . Age Ageing, 37(1, 19–24. .

Schmalzl, L., Crane-Godreau, M. A., & and Payne, P. (2014). Movement-based embodied contemplative practices: definitions and paradigms. Front Hum Neurosci.; 8: 205.

ScienceDirect. (2018). Available at: https://www.sciencedirect.com/topics/neuroscience/visual-system. Accessed on June30.

Shumway-Cook A, W. M. (2007). Motor Control Translating Research Into Clinical Practice. 3rd ed Philadelphia, PA: Lippincott Williams & Wilkins.

Stanford University, T. C. (2018). The History of Tai Chi Chuan. Available at: https://web.stanford.edu/group/taichi_wushu/taichi.history.html. Acessed on May 18.

Sungkarat S, B. S. (2018). Tai Chi Improves Cognition and Plasma BDNF in Older Adults With Mild Cognitive Impairment: A Randomized Controlled Trial. Neurorehabil Neural Repair. Feb;32 (2), 142-149.

Suzuki, S. (1970). Zen Mind, Beginner's Mind. New York, NY: Weatherhill.

Swenson, R. (2018). Chapter 7E -Vestibular System. Available at: https://www.dartmouth.edu/~rswenson/NeuroSci/chapter_7E.html. Accessed on Jun 30.

(2018). Tai Chi Clothing. Available at: http://taichibasics.com/tai-chi-clothing/. Accessed on July, 08.

Taichicentral.com. (2018). History of Tai Chi. Available at: https://taichicentral.com/about-tai-chi/history-of-tai-chi/. Acessed on May 27, 2018.

Tao J, L. J. (2017). Tai Chi Chuan and Baduanjin Increase Grey Matter Volume in Older Adults: A Brain Imaging Study. J Alzheimers Dis. 60 (2), 389-400.

Teahupoo. (2018). Why Proper Clothing Is So Important In Tai Chi. Availableat: http://www.streetdirectory.com/travel_guide/22961/modelling/why_proper_clothing_is_so_important_in_tai_chi.html. Accessed on June 10.

(2018). The history of Tai Chi. Available at: http://www.seas.ucla.edu/spapl/qifeng/history.html. Acessed on May 17.

(2018). The History of Tai Chi. Available at: http://www.kienandokungfu.com/Tai_Chi_Chuan.htm. Acessed on May 26, 2018.

Toosizadeh, N., Ehsani, H., Miramonte, M., & and Mohler, J. (2018). Proprioceptive impairments in high fall risk older adults: the effect of mechanical calf vibration on postural balance. Biomed Eng Online; 17: 51.

Tsai PF1, K. S. (2017). hi for Posttraumatic Stress Disorder and Chronic Musculoskeletal Pain: A Pilot Study. J Holist Nurs. Mar .

Tsai, P. F. (2013). A pilot cluster-randomized trial of a 20-week Tai Chi program in elders with cognitive impairment and osteoarthritic knee: effects on pain and other health outcomes. . J Pain Symptom Manage. 45, 660–669.

Vitetta, L. A. (2005). Mind-body medicine: stress and its impact on overall health and longevity. Ann N Y Acad, 492–505 .

Wang F, L. E. (2014). The effects of tai chi on depression, anxiety, and psychological well-being: a systematic review and meta-analysis. Int J Behav Med. Aug;21 (4), 605-17.

Wang, C. e. (2009). Tai Chi is effective in treating knee osteoarthritis: a randomized controlled trial. Arthritis Rheum. 61, 1545–1553.

Was Confucianism a Religion or Philosophy? . (2018). Available at: https://www.essaytown.com/subjects/paper/confucianism-religion-philosophy/7080669. Accesed on May 26.

What is Tao? (2018). Available at: http://www.bbc.co.uk/religion/religions/taoism/beliefs/tao.shtml. Accessed on May 25, 2018.

WHO, W. H. (2018). Constitution of WHO: principles. Available at: Constitution of WHO: principles. Accessed on July 02.

WHO, W. H. (2018). WHO Global Report on Falls Prevention in Older Age. Accessed on April 16, 2108. Available at: http://www.who.int/ageing/publications/Falls_prevention7March.pdf?ua=1.

Wikipedia. (2018). Anatomical plane. Available at: https://en.wikipedia.org/wiki/Anatomical_plane. Accessed on Jun 30.

Wikipedia. (2018). Bagua. Available at: https://en.wikipedia.org/wiki/Bagua. Accessed on May 27.

Wikipedia. (2018). Wu-style t'ai chi ch'uan. Available at: https://en.wikipedia.org/wiki/Wu-style_t%27ai_chi_ch%27uan. Accessed on Jun 02.

Wile, D. (1995). Lost T'ai-chi Classics from the Late Ch'ing Dynasty (Chinese Philosophy and Culture). State University of New York Press.

Wilhelm, R. (. (1967). The I Ching or Book of Changes. translated by Cary F. Baynes, forward by C. G. Jung, preface to 3rd ed. by Hellmut Wilhelm. Princeton, NJ: Princeton University Press.

Yang-style t'ai chi ch'uan. (2018, Avaliable at: https://en.wikipedia.org/wiki/Yang-style_t%27ai_chi_ch%27uan. Accessed on May 05).

Yip, L. (April, 1998). "Principles and Practice of Sun Style T'ai Chi – T'AI CHI The International Magazine of T'ai Chi Ch'uan. Vol. 22 No. 2". Wayfarer Publications.

Yip, Y. L. (Autumn 2002). "Pivot". Qi, The Journal of Traditional Eastern Health and Fitness. Insight Graphics Publishers.

Zhi-Guan Huang, Y.-H. F.-H.-S. (2017). Systematic review and meta-analysis: Tai Chi for preventing falls in older adults. BMJ Open 7:e013661. .

Zimi Ma, C. J. (2014). Features analysis of five-element theory and its basal effects on construction. Journal of Traditional Chinease Medicine, February 15; 34(1): 115-121.

Bibliography Consulted

Ancient Way to Keep Fit, by Zong Wu and Li Mao, 1992, pp. 68-80.

Seong-Dae Woo, Tae-Ho Kim, Jin-Yong Lim. The effects of breathing with mainly inspiration or expiration on pulmonary function and chest expansion. J. Phys. Ther. Sci. 28: 927–931, 2016

K Rajeshwari , Shivani Kohli , Xavier K Mathew. Evaluation of Resting Tongue Position in Recently Extracted and Long Term Completely Edentulous Patients: A Prospective Interventional Study. Journal of Clinical and Diagnostic Research. 2017 Apr, Vol-11(4): ZC61-ZC63

Park SY. Sleep Apnea Is a Craniofacial Problem. http://doctorstevenpark.com/sleep-apnea-is-a-craniofacial-problem.

Published February 10, 2011. Accessed May 27, 2016.

Hanson ML, Mason RM. Orofacial Myology: International Perspectives. 2nd ed. Springfield, IL: Charles C Thomas; 2003.

Proffit WR. Equilibrium Theory Revisited: Factors Influencing Position of the Teeth. Angle Orthod. 1978;48(3):175-186.
Shanti McGinley. The Roles of Oral Rest Posture and Neutral Position in Articulation Therapy. Available at: https://pammarshalla.com/the-roles-of-oral-rest-posture-and-neutral-position-in-articulation-therapy/
Chen, Jinhua (2007). Philosopher, Practitioner, Politician: The Many Lives of Fazang (643-712). Brill.
Proffit WR. Equilibrium Theory Revisited: Factors Influencing Position of the Teeth. Angle Orthod. 1978;48(3):175-186.
Mason RM, Franklin H. Orofacial Myofunctional Disorders and Otolaryngologists. Otolaryng. 2014; 4:e100.
A Source Book in Chinese Longevity. By Livia Kohn. University Of Hawaii Press
Chinese Healing Exercises: The Tradition of Daoyin. By Livia Kohn. University Of Hawaii Press.

www.ingramcontent.com/pod-product-compliance
Lightning Source LLC
Chambersburg PA
CBHW051501050726
47593CB00005B/2164